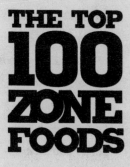

THE TOP
100
ZONE
FOODS

By Dr. Barry Sears

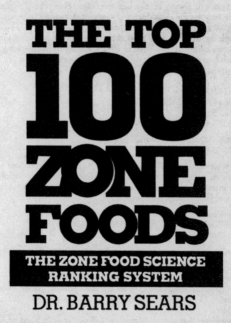

THE TOP
100
ZONE
FOODS

THE ZONE FOOD SCIENCE RANKING SYSTEM

DR. BARRY SEARS

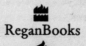

ReganBooks

HarperTorch
An Imprint of HarperCollins*Publishers*

This book is not intended to replace medical advice or to be a substitute for a physician. If you are sick or suspect you are sick, you should see a physician. If you are taking a prescription medication, you should never change your diet (for better or worse) without consulting your physician, because any dietary change will affect the metabolism of that prescription drug.

Prevention will always be the best medicine. However, prevention can be undertaken only by the individual, and that includes eating correctly. This is the foundation of a healthy lifestyle. You have to eat, so you may as well eat wisely.

Although this book is about food, the author and the publisher expressly disclaim responsibility for any adverse effects arising from following the advice given in this book without appropriate medical supervision.

HARPERTORCH
An Imprint of HarperCollins*Publishers*
10 East 53rd Street
New York, New York 10022-5299

Copyright © 2001 by Barry Sears, Ph.D.
ISBN: 0-06-074185-6

First HarperTorch/ReganBooks paperback printing: January 2005
First ReganBooks trade paperback printing: January 2002
First ReganBooks hardcover printing: January 2001

The ReganBooks hardcover edition contains the following Library of Congress Cataloging-in-Publication Data:

Sears, Barry, 1947–
    The top 100 zone foods : the zone food science ranking system / Barry Sears.
        p.   cm.
Includes index.
1. Reducing diets—Recipes. 2. Nutrition. I. Title: Top one hundred Zone foods.
II. Title.
RM222.2.S3895 2001
613.2—dc21   00-045886

Contents

Appendixes

Acknowledgments

The success of the Zone books that I have written during the past five years is primarily due to my team who is not only my co-workers, but also my closest friends. These include my wife, Lynn Sears, who does much of the editing of my books, and my brother, Doug Sears, who has a very clear insight and understanding of how to translate cutting-edge science into easily understood terms for the general public. In addition, I wish to especially thank Deborah Kotz for her excellent advice and editorial input in helping develop this book.

Special thanks go to Roberto Mighty and Joseph Alsop, who orchestrated the various recipes to illustrate how easy it is to incorporate the Top 100 Zone Foods into great Zone meals.

At the same time, I also have my team at ReganBooks who consistently do an outstanding job of fine-tuning my books for the general public. For this particular book, I want to give special thanks to Doug Corcoran for his excellent editing.

Of course, my greatest thanks always goes to Judith Regan, who had the courage and foresight to support the Zone, and in the process helped improve the lives of millions of people.

Introduction

Since the dawn of time, scientific discoveries have been ridiculed and violently rejected before they became self-evident. Galileo was imprisoned for asserting that the earth revolved around the sun. Columbus was laughed at for suggesting that the earth was round. As with all innovative discoveries, the Zone has pretty much followed the same course. When I first came up with the concept of the Zone some twenty years ago, my idea was strongly ridiculed, and I was labeled as a charlatan. The publication of my first book, *The Zone,* more than five years ago generated a firestorm of criticism often bordering on irrational vehemence.

As we settle into the twenty-first century, the Zone is on the verge of becoming a mainstream nutritional program. I get more and more letters from physicians who tell me they prescribe the Zone to their patients, and I hear more nutritionists grudgingly admit that the Zone is a reasonable diet. Some of my most vociferous past critics are now adopting many of the concepts of the Zone as their own. I welcome such a growing consensus. As the old saying goes, victory has a thousand fathers.

I'm not surprised that the Zone has been embraced by millions. After all, the program is based on simple dietary common sense: balance and moderation. I'm not trying to sell you a bill of goods by saying you can eat as much steak or cheesecake as you want. What I'm giving you is intuitive dietary wisdom based on cutting-edge science. Simply balance your plate with protein and carbohydrates, add a dash of fat, and eat only a moderate number of total calories at each meal. The end result? Better hormonal control, specifically keeping the hormone insulin within a zone that is neither too high nor too low.

As the majority of Americans struggle with obesity, the concepts of balance and moderation have been thrown out the window. You may think that the "answer" to this obesity epidemic lies in an extreme diet. In fact, you may have tried one yourself: the high-protein diet of steak and eggs or the high-carbohydrate "bagel" diet. The Zone is not high-anything, because it's based on balance, the very thing that your body needs to function at its best.

The goal of this book is to get you to feel the beneficial effects of the Zone and to give you the tools to prepare the very best possible Zone meals. You will learn how to incorporate the highest-quality foods you can find into the Zone Diet. The payoff is huge: You'll get the greatest potential control over your insulin levels, which means a lower risk of heart disease, diabetes, and cancer. You'll get the additional benefit of losing those stubborn fat pounds that you've never been able to get rid of in the past.

As I said, I'm not trying to sell you an unproven theory. These hefty promises are backed by solid science. If you're already aware of the Zone Diet, you know that it's based on research that has determined the ratio of carbohydrates, fat, and protein you need to get the hormonal response that sends you into the Zone.

This book takes the Zone Diet and combines it with a new Zone Food Science Ranking System that I developed using mathematical formulas to evaluate the quality of the foods we eat. Using these formulas, I identified the Top 100 highest-quality foods you should eat when following the Zone Diet. Like high-octane gasoline, these high-quality foods are the very best fuel you can put in your body. Yes, you can make a Zone meal out of low-octane foods—like a few pieces of salami on a slice of white bread. But you'll get the maximum hormonal mileage out of every meal if you choose high-octane foods like grilled tuna accompanied by an assortment of free-radical-fighting vegetables and fruits. You're probably already including some of these Top 100 foods in your current diet, but you'll also see how easy it is to include new foods from the list that you've never tried.

All you really need to keep in mind is the ultimate goal of the Zone: lifelong hormonal control. Once you become the master of your hormones, you can halt or even reverse the aging process. You'll retain muscle mass (which naturally declines as you age), avoid those inevitable old-age ailments like heart disease, cancer, and arthritis, and even prevent wrinkles. This book will teach you how easy it is to treat food with the same respect as any prescription drug, while at the same time enhancing the pleasure you get from every bite you take. In fact, many people with adult-onset diabetes (Type 2 diabetes) have been able to use the Zone to completely control their disease without any medications, including insulin injections. Other Zone advocates have been able to go off the blood pressure or cholesterol-lowering drugs their doctors had told them they would have to use for the rest of their lives. I'd much rather eat a savory piece of salmon covered with crisp vegetables than swallow a bitter pill with numerous side effects. Wouldn't you? If you choose food as your health elixir for the future, then this book is written expressly for you. Welcome to the Zone!

Making the Top 100

You probably assume you're a product of your genes. You have your father's eyes, your mother's freckles, and your grandmother's diabetes. I, too, am a product of my genes. Every male on my father's side has died an early death after suffering a premature heart attack. My father died in 1972 at the age of 54, and I was sure that I was genetically destined for this same fate.

Although I knew I couldn't change my genes, I didn't want to be a slave to them either. I was determined to alter my genetic destiny and live a normal, healthy lifespan. I didn't buy into the notion that some new medication would come along to save me. I had to take charge of my own health directly by changing my eating habits. So I decided to devote my work as a researcher to discovering what, if any, dietary habits could reverse my impending collision course with my genetic fate. Through 20 years of research, I've learned that food can indirectly turn certain genes on and off by altering the levels of hormones, the chemical messengers that control our lives. These hormones can alter our genetic fate by increasing or decreasing our natural lifespan.

One of the most powerful hormones controlled by the foods we eat is insulin. My research found that if you could keep insulin levels within a certain zone—not too high and not too low—you could, in fact, bypass your genetic glitches and avoid certain chronic diseases. The result? A longer and healthier life.

I called my program the Zone Diet. Although it was developed for treating cardiovascular disease and Type 2 diabetes, it is also the most effective way to lose excess body fat without feeling deprived or hungry. It is not a short-term diet, but a life-long dietary strategy that can keep you at a healthy weight for the rest of your life. All you need to do is eat the right combination of foods at every meal. This means eating a balanced amount of carbohydrates, protein, and fat at every meal and snack—and eating all these foods in moderation. Follow this simple rule at every meal, and you will achieve the hormonal responses that will get you into the Zone.

What does it mean to be in the Zone? Picture yourself going through your days feeling energized, happy, and satisfied. That's the feeling you get in the Zone. Now picture yourself feeling exhausted, hungry, and down in the dumps. That's what you feel like when you're out of the Zone. If you follow my Zone prescription, within a week you will be thinking better, performing better, and looking better. In the long run, you'll receive some rather remarkable health benefits like the permanent loss of excess body fat and a dramatically lowered risk of diabetes and heart disease.

The Zone has been incorrectly dubbed a high-protein diet by the popular press. The Zone is not a high-protein, high-carbohydrate, or high-anything diet. These diets are faddish quick fixes and run contrary to what Nature intended. The Zone is a balanced diet in the truest sense of the word. To stay healthy, you need to keep all of your body's systems in balance, and that's what the Zone Diet will do for you.

THE HEALTHIEST DIET IN THE WORLD

I firmly believe that the Zone Diet is the healthiest diet in the world. Like any piece of technology, the Zone keeps evolving. When I first created the Zone, I came up with a system called Zone Food Blocks and divided all foods into various blocks of protein, carbohydrate, and fat so that you could mix and match them to get the best hormonal output. As long as you have the right combination of protein, carbohydrate, and fat blocks, you can achieve the hormonal effects of the Zone. You do, however, still need to be selective about the quality of foods you eat. I also told you to avoid certain carbohydrates that cause dangerous rises in insulin (like bagels and potatoes). Dining on low-fat protein, heart-healthy fats, and tons of fruits and vegetables makes the Zone Diet the hands-down most nutritious eating plan you can follow.

The Zone Diet has continued to evolve into increasingly healthier versions; such as replacing low-fat animal protein with increasing amounts of soy protein. I wrote *The Soy Zone* based on the diet eaten by the longest-living population in the world, the Okinawans. Their basic diet is the Zone Diet, containing primarily vegetables, some fish and animal protein, but with most of their protein from soy. That's why you'll find numerous soy protein products on my Top 100 list.

For this book I took a little journey down memory lane. I went back through all my years of research and searched through studies conducted by other scientists to determine which particular foods are the absolute best for your health. New information is coming along every day, but all the foods on my Top 100 list have been found to have significant health benefits in study after study.

Of course, I'm not telling you that you need to eat only these foods. I want you to experience the hundreds of varieties of fruits and vegetables whose shimmering colors catch your eye on produce stands. (As you will find out later, more color means more free-radical-fighting abilities.) I do, however, think it's important to make certain foods staples in your diet. For instance, you can follow the Zone Diet and never eat a single cruciferous vegetable, yet you'd be missing out on the cancer- and aging-fighting chemicals that make broccoli, spinach, and kale so potent in lowering the risk of heart disease and cancer.

If you aren't using the highest-quality foods in your Zone meals, then you aren't reaping the maximum health benefits of the Zone. It's as simple as that. Maybe you're not quite sure how to fit your favorite fruits and vegetables into the plan. Perhaps you're reluctant to try something new if you don't have a recipe to use it in. Chapter 4, "The Top 100 Zone Foods," will give you easy and delicious recipes containing all of these foods.

These 100 foods are the highest-quality foods you can get. They were the ones that came up on top when I put thousands of foods through my Zone Food Science Ranking System. I believe they will help you achieve the peak effects of the Zone by giving you the biggest bang for the buck.

The point is to get you to incorporate as many of the foods as possible into your Zone eating plan—not just the healthiest five foods on each list. I want you to get out of the tomato-cucumber-lettuce salad rut. By the time you're through with this book, you won't think twice about mixing some orange slices with some spinach leaves to create a salad or tossing some chickpeas in with your steamed broccoli.

I want to get you out of the "if it's Tuesday, it must be chicken" mindset and into the "variety, variety, variety" mode. That's the message of the U.S. government and the American Heart Association when they tell you to eat 3 to 5 servings of fruits and vegetables a day. (The Zone Diet actually surpasses this by recommending 10 to 15 servings per day.) Each food on my Top 100 list contains its own array of disease-fighting chemicals that help keep your body healthy. Combine these foods according to Zone principles, and you've covered all your bases. Your body will have all the nutrients it needs and will have a full arsenal of weapons at its disposal to fight disease and live a longer and better life.

To qualify for my Top 100 list, the Zone foods have to meet two criteria:

1. They have to be nutrient-dense.
2. They have to work the most effectively to improve your insulin levels, enabling you to enter the Zone and stay there on a long-term basis.

Use these foods identified by the Zone Food Science Ranking System, and you have the quickest and most effective way to get yourself into the Zone.

INSTANT GRATIFICATION IN THE ZONE

If you've never entered the Zone, you'll be amazed at how great you feel once you're there. Within one week in the Zone, you will:

- **Get mentally focused.** Keeping your blood sugar level on an even keel throughout the day, you'll find you have a better ability to concentrate and won't have that mental haziness that can strike two to three hours after eating a high-carbohydrate meal.

- **Experience a surge of energy.** Adding more (but not too much) protein to your diet will increase your levels of the hormone glucagon, which helps your body maintain constant blood sugar levels for mental energy. Once you lower your insulin levels, you can access your stored body fat for an almost inexhaustible source of energy for increased physical activity. You'll find yourself operating at peak performance throughout the day. Afternoon mental slumps will be a thing of the past. Coming home, you'll have the excess energy to enjoy life to its fullest.

- **Lose a few pounds of fat.** You'll see a change in your body shape as you begin to shed fat. You can expect to lose up to 5 pounds during your first week on the Zone Diet (1 to 2 pounds of fat and 2 to 3 pounds of retained water). Excess insulin levels generated by high-carbohydrate diets cause you to retain 2 to 3 pounds of water that are shed once you switch to fewer carbohydrates and more protein.

- **Feel happier.** The sugar lows that leave you feeling tired, hungry, and irritable between meals will be banished for good. You'll no longer feel like a slave to food and will no longer be plagued by carbohydrate cravings. Overall, your body will feel like a well-tuned machine, a sign that your hormones are in tune, too.

- **Gain control over your insulin levels.** Several studies have shown that within hours of going on the

Zone Diet, people experience a reduction in excess insulin levels, the underlying cause of diabetes and heart disease. A recent study from Harvard Medical School found that the insulin-controlling benefits kick in after just one meal in the Zone. (Of course, your insulin levels will shoot right back up if you have a meal that's not Zone balanced.)

If you follow the Zone Diet, you'll experience all these benefits just by making a few simple changes in your eating habits. Of course these are great short-term benefits, but the real reason you want to make the Zone an integral part of your life is that it can improve your health dramatically and will lead to a longer life.

By incorporating the Top 100 Zone Foods into your Zone eating plan, you will maximize the long-term health effects of the Zone. Getting the proper balance of protein, carbohydrates, and fat will take you most of the way there. Adding the highest-quality foods in each of these categories will allow you to reap the full benefits of the Zone. Living a healthier life will allow you to lead a fuller and happier life—and isn't that the point of it all?

A vast number of health benefits can result simply from getting better control of your insulin levels. In the Zone:

1. **You will achieve permanent fat loss.** The best way to get a handle on your weight is to control your insulin levels. Through the Zone, you will naturally shed all the body fat that your body doesn't need. Many Zone users have lost 20, 40, or in some cases more than 100 pounds. More important, they have kept those pounds off over the years.

2. **You will reduce your risk of heart disease.** As you lower your insulin levels, you will also lower your

likelihood of heart disease. A study reported in the *Journal of the American Medical Association* found that insulin levels are far more predictive for the development of heart disease than any other risk factor.

3. **You will protect yourself against adult-onset (Type 2) diabetes.** In this type of diabetes (which accounts for more than 90 percent of all cases), people produce too much insulin, which can destroy healthy organs and tissues in the body. Clinical studies have shown that the Zone lowers excess insulin levels in Type 2 diabetics within four days.

4. **You will lower your risk of arthritis and osteoporosis.** Lowering insulin can alleviate tissue inflammation, because reduced insulin levels also mean reduced levels of the building blocks of pain-producing eicosanoids. By decreasing these types of eicosanoids, you relieve the pain and inflammation associated with arthritis. Research has also shown that increased protein consumption actually decreases the number of hip fractures in postmenopausal women.

5. **You may reduce your risk of developing breast cancer.** A number of studies have found an association between high insulin levels and increased risk of breast cancer. What's more, research from Harvard Medical School has shown that the more protein (and fewer carbohydrates) a woman consumes, the better her survival rate after breast cancer.

6. **You'll get fewer infections.** Adequate protein ensures proper functioning of the immune system, the body's natural defense mechanism against disease. Many people on high-carbohydrate diets have suppressed immune systems and are more susceptible to infection because of excess insulin levels. They're

more likely to get sick (not to mention catching
colds and the flu) than people getting adequate protein throughout the day.

7. **Your skin will look younger.** The primary cause of
wrinkles in the skin is inflammation in the skin. Reduce this inflammation by eating anti-oxidant-rich
carbohydrates and cutting back on Omega-6 fats
(such as safflower, corn, and soybean oils) and
you'll be able to prevent wrinkles and other signs of
skin aging.

All of these bold promises can be fulfilled if you
combine the Zone Diet plan with the Top 100 Zone
Foods outlined in Chapter 4. Once you understand the
basic rules of the Zone and how I came to pick the
foods for my Top 100 list, you'll be ready to dive into
the recipes.

Your Zone Primer

To enter the Zone, you need to learn how to maintain the hormones produced by the foods you eat within a Zone (not too high, not too low). These hormones are readjusted every time you eat a meal or snack, so you're only as good or as bad as your last meal. This means that if you splurge and eat too many carbohydrates in one sitting, you can get back into the Zone the next time you eat. Thus you don't need to feel guilty about cheating. Just make your next meal Zone-friendly.

The Zone is not some clever marketing phrase. The Zone has a very precise medical definition that can be measured with a simple blood test. The next time you have a blood test, ask your doctor to measure your fasting insulin levels. If your insulin levels are too high (greater than 10 uU/ml), you know that you're not in the Zone. The sluggishness, hunger, and moodiness you feel in between meals are all signs that you're out of the Zone.

You can lower your insulin levels to get into the Zone. The only "drug" that can take you there is food. In the process, you'll radically improve your quality of life. You'll feel less tired, more mentally charged, and happier throughout the day. Your new hormonal balance will be giving your body the continuous fuel it needs to keep all your systems operating at their peak performance. You will feel your body telling you that "all systems are go" and that the possibilities of what you can do are limitless.

How can you gain control of your unruly hormones? You need to wipe away many of the nutrition myths that you've probably come to believe—for example, that fat is bad and pasta is good. You need to stop fooling yourself into thinking that you can lose weight while eating fat-free cookies or fat-free ice cream. You need to embrace the notion that you must have a balance of the three major categories of food (protein, carbohydrates, and fat) at every meal to get the right response from your body.

You also need to be selective about the *quality* of the foods you choose within each category to get the most hormonal cluck for your buck. For instance, fried bacon with hash browns won't give you as good a hormonal response as grilled chicken breast with asparagus and green beans with fresh fruit for dessert. Get the right balance and quality of foods, and your body will produce the appropriate hormonal signals for the next four to six hours. During this time, you will be in the Zone. You can keep yourself there by eating the same balance of foods at your next meal or snack. But you still need to be selective about the quality of foods you choose within each category.

THE RATIONALE BEHIND MY TOP 100 LIST

I want you to think about food as an exceptionally powerful drug that contains protein, carbohydrates, and fat. All foods are composed of these three "macronutrients" to varying degrees. Most foods contain a bulk of one group and trace amounts of the others. In a nutshell, protein includes all things that move around, like fish, fowl, and cattle. Carbohydrates consist of things that grow in the ground, like wheat, potatoes, and, yes, fruits and vegetables. The fact that fruits and vegetables are carbohydrates may come as a revelation to you. Finally, fats are found in both animal products and plant oils. One reason you may be so confused about eating is that you don't fully understand what you are eating.

All carbohydrates are not created equal. Neither are all proteins or all fats. This is just common sense. You know that an apple is much healthier than a piece of chocolate cake, and your body knows it, too. It does not treat all carbohydrates the same, and it knows how to distinguish between the types of fat and protein as well. The types of foods you eat can have dramatically different effects on hormones such as insulin. So it's not enough to get the right combination of carbohydrates, fats, and proteins. You need to eat the right kinds of these foods. You need to go for high-quality foods and avoid low-quality ones.

Those foods I identified as the most nutritious foods you can put in your body appear on my list of Top 100 Zone Foods. If you incorporate these foods into the Zone Diet, you will indeed be eating the healthiest diet in the world.

To create my Top 100 list, I tapped into the U.S. Department of Agriculture (USDA) Nutrient Databases and used it to help determine the best choices. As you will see later in the book, the results may be surprising, since many of the foods that the government recommends are actually pretty poor choices for any diet, let alone the Zone Diet.

LEARNING THE BASIC RULES OF THE ZONE: THE HAND-EYE METHOD

Once you think of foods in terms of their three major categories, you can easily master the basic rules of the Zone. How can you use carbohydrates, protein, and fat to get yourself into the Zone? Just follow the common-sense approach your grandmother taught you: *balance* and *moderation*. Balance your plate at every meal, and never eat too many calories at any meal. The only tools you need are the palm of your hand and your eye—which is why I call this the hand-eye method.

Step #1: Start with Protein

Every Zone meal and snack starts with an adequate serving of low-fat protein. The protein category of the Top 100 list contains the highest-quality protein choices. High-quality protein means that it is low in heart-damaging saturated fat and high in nutrients like zinc or calcium. Dark-fleshed fish (like salmon and tuna) also make it to the Top 100 list because they contain long-chain Omega-3 fats, which can protect your heart and increase your lifespan, as I have detailed in my other books. Soy protein ranks high on the Top 100 list because it can lower insulin levels even more than other types of animal protein.

Your body needs a constant supply of dietary protein to replace the protein that is lost from your body on a daily basis. What's more, eating protein stimulates the release of the hormone glucagon, which has a hormonal effect opposite to that of insulin. Glucagon tells your body to release stored carbohydrates from the liver to replenish blood sugar levels in the brain. Without adequate levels of glucagon, you'll always feel hungry and mentally fatigued because your brain is short on its primary fuel—blood sugar.

The first step of Zone meal preparation is never to consume any more low-fat protein than you can fit in the palm of your hand or that is any thicker than your hand. For the average American female, this amount is 3 ounces of low-fat protein, and for the average American male it is about 4 ounces. Unless you are active, your body can't utilize any more protein than that at a single sitting, and any excess protein will be converted to fat.

Divide your plate into three portions. Your low-fat protein portion should cover about one-third of your plate.

Step #2: Balance with Carbohydrates

Once you have the protein portion of your meal, you need to balance it with carbohydrates. Remember: fruits and vegetables are carbohydrates. In fact, they are the highest-quality carbohydrates you can eat, which is why (with one or two exceptions) they are the only carbohydrates you'll find on my Top 100 list. The reason you won't find pasta, rice, or mashed potatoes on my list is that they wreak havoc on your body without providing much nutrition. First of all, these carbohydrates cause dangerous spikes in your insulin levels, which cause your blood sugar levels to rise and then quickly fall, leaving you famished just two hours after eating. Second, these carbohydrates contain very few vitamins and minerals (unless they're artificially fortified) and only sparse amounts of phytochemicals, the tiny plant chemicals that can ward off cancer, heart disease, and other illnesses by acting as powerful anti-oxidants.

On the other hand, fruits and vegetables meet both

of my criteria for high-quality foods. They are packed with natural vitamins, minerals, and phytochemicals. They also contain fiber, which slows the release of insulin so you won't get quick spikes in your blood sugar. This is why an apple leaves you feeling satisfied longer than a cookie. Not all carbohydrates are equal in their ability to stimulate the production of insulin. The high-quality carbohydrates are favorable in that they have a low capacity to stimulate insulin; others are unfavorable in that they have a high capacity to stimulate insulin. You'll find only favorable carbohydrates on my Top 100 list.

Your high-quality carbohydrate portion should cover the other two-thirds of your plate.

Step #3: Add Fat

Now your plate is completely covered. Protein takes up one-third of the space, and carbohydrates take up the other two-thirds. Where does fat fit in? Fat is the sprinkling that seasons your foods—whether it's the teaspoon of olive oil that you cook your vegetables in or the avocado slices or handful of slivered almonds that you add to your salads. Without fat, you can't have a complete Zone meal.

Fat has no direct effect on insulin, nor does it have any effect on glucagon. Fat, though, acts like a control rod in a nuclear reactor, slowing the rate at which carbohydrates enter your bloodstream. In addition, it also causes the release of another hormone that tells your brain to stop eating. Finally, fat gives you a feeling of satiety and helps blend the flavors that give great meals their exquisite taste.

The high-quality fats that make my Top 100 list are those that are good for your heart and your health in general. These are the monounsaturated fats and long-chain Omega-3 fats. You get monounsaturated fats from olive oil, selected nuts, and avocados. Long-chain Omega-3 fats come from fish and fish oils (like the cod liver oil your grandmother told you to take). These are exceptionally powerful allies in your quest for a longer life.

The fats that are absent from my Top 100 are the saturated fats, trans fats, and Omega-6 fats. You find saturated fats in fatty cuts of red meat and high-fat dairy products. You find trans fats in margarine and other partially hydrogenated oils found in many processed snack foods. Polyunsaturated fats like corn and safflower oil are rich in Omega-6 fats, which in excess are far worse for you hormonally than saturated fats. I consider these Omega-6 fats to be the really "bad" fats because they can lead to increased inflammation, which is an underlying cause of heart disease and arthritis.

Add a dash (that's a small amount) of "good" fat to complete your Zone plate.

A QUICK REVIEW OF YOUR ZONE PLATE

Now that you have an idea what types of protein, carbohydrate, and fat you will be using to make Zone meals and snacks, let me show you how easy it really is.

Just divide your plate into three sections. On one-third of your plate, choose one of the protein choices from my Top 100 Zone Foods list—no bigger than the size and thickness of your palm. Then fill the other two-thirds of the plate until it is overflowing with the carbohydrate choices from the Top 100. Add a sprinkling of fat from the choices in the fat category. There you have it: a Zone meal.

I use the term *meal* loosely. On the Zone Diet, you should be eating three meals a day and two snacks. When composing your meals, use a dinner-size plate. When composing your snacks, use a dessert plate. It couldn't be any easier.

**Divide Your Plate
Into 3 Sections.**

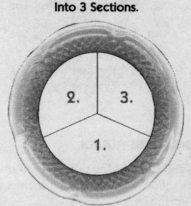

Start with Low-Fat Protein . . .

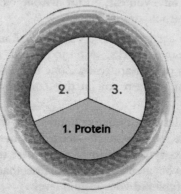

**Fill other sections with vegetables
and some fruits.**

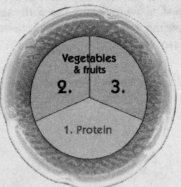

THE BASIC ZONE RULES

Now that you know what goes into your Zone meal,
you need to follow a few other simple rules to get in the
Zone and stay there.

1. Always eat a Zone meal within one hour after waking.
2. Every time you eat, go for a Zone balance of pro-
    tein, carbohydrates, and fat.
3. Try to eat five times a day: three Zone meals and
    two Zone snacks. Afternoon and late evening
    snacks (which are really Zone mini-meals) are im-
    portant to keep you in the Zone throughout the
    day.
4. Never let more than five hours go by without eating
    a Zone meal or snack—regardless of whether you
    are hungry or not. In fact, the best time to eat is
    when you aren't hungry because that means you
    have stabilized your insulin levels.

5. Eat more fruits and vegetables (yes, these are car-
    bohydrates) and ease off the bread, pasta, grains,
    and other starches. Treat these low-quality carbo-
    hydrates like condiments.

6. Drink at least eight 8-ounce glasses of water every
    day.

7. If you make a mistake at a meal, don't worry about
    it. There's no guilt in the Zone. Just make your next
    meal a Zone meal to get you where you (and your
    hormones) belong.

A DAY IN THE ZONE

Now that you know the basic Zone rules, let's see what
a typical day in the Zone for a typical American female
might look like. These foods are all found on my Top
100 list.

Breakfast

A six-egg-white omelette mixed with some asparagus
and 2 teaspoons of olive oil; ⅔ cup of slow-cooked oatmeal; and a cup of strawberries.

Lunch

Orange, tofu, and spinach salad: 1 pound of baby
spinach leaves mixed with orange slices and 4½ ounces
of smoked tofu, topped with plum vinegar and 1⅓ teaspoons of sesame oil; a piece of fruit for dessert.

Late-Afternoon Snack

Two hard-boiled eggs with the yolks removed and replaced with hummus (mashed chickpeas and olive oil).

Dinner

A 5-ounce piece of salmon covered with a tablespoon of slivered almonds; three cups of steamed vegetables; a cup of mixed berries for dessert.

Late-Night Snack

A 1-ounce piece of soft low-fat cheese and a glass of wine (or a small piece of fruit if you don't drink).

Just glancing through this, you should notice that it's a lot of food. That's because you're eating low-density carbohydrates in the form of fruits and vegetables. On a volume basis, fruits and vegetables contain much fewer carbohydrates than high-density bread and pasta. This means you get more food in fewer calories. For this reason, women typically eat only about 1,200 calories a day on the Zone and men only about 1,500 calories per day. This is what I call the Zone paradox. You can consume a lot of food without getting a lot of calories or feeling hungry or deprived. You will also lose weight, which is an added plus. Most importantly, if you eat only Zone meals and snacks, you are greatly increasing your chance for a longer life by keeping your overall calorie count at a level that has been shown by 60 years of research to be the only way to reach your maximum longevity.

ZONE MEAL TIMING

Meal timing is critically important for staying in the Zone, just as it is in taking a drug. Set a beeper alarm on your watch to remind yourself to eat if you have to.

I can't emphasize enough how vital it is to eat five times a day (three meals and two snacks). A typical meal schedule might be as follows: If you wake up at 6:00 A.M., you should eat a Zone breakfast by 7:00. (This is a substantial breakfast, not a piece of toast on the run.) Five hours later, it's noon and time for lunch, which will be another big meal. Most people won't eat dinner before 7:00 P.M., which is more than five hours after lunch, so have a snack in the late afternoon. After eating dinner at 7:00, make sure you have one final late-night snack before you go to bed, because your brain still needs blood sugar during your eight hours of sleep. That's your typical day in the Zone.

Timing of Zone Meals

Meal	Timing	Approximate Time
Breakfast	Within 1 hour after waking	7:00 A.M.
Lunch	Within 5 hours after breakfast	12:00 P.M.
Late-afternoon snack	Within 5 hours after lunch	5:00 P.M
Dinner	Within 2–3 hours after snack	7:00 P.M.
Late-night snack	Before bed	11:00 P.M.

FINE-TUNING THE ZONE DIET

You may find that creating Zone meals using the hand-eye method described earlier in the chapter works well to get you into the Zone. Some people don't like to estimate portion sizes, however, and would prefer a more scientific way of measuring out carbohydrates, protein, and fat. If you are one of these people, you should consider using the Zone Food Block method.

The Zone Food Block method gives you a sense of greater dietary control, but it gives you virtually the same results as the hand-eye method. Instead of using your plate as a guide, you'll be counting out blocks of protein, carbohydrates, and fat. One Zone Food Block of protein contains 7 grams of protein, and the average woman will need three Protein Blocks for each meal (about 20 grams of protein). The average man requires four Zone Protein Blocks (about 30 grams of protein). This translates into about 3 ounces of high-quality protein for a woman and about 4 ounces of high-quality protein for a man.

Now it's time to balance your protein with an appropriate amount of carbohydrates. You need to eat the same number of Zone Carbohydrate Blocks at every meal as Protein Blocks. Thus if you need three Protein Blocks, you should also eat three Carbohydrate Blocks. One Carbohydrate Block contains 9 grams, so you should be getting 27 grams of carbohydrates in three blocks and 36 grams in four blocks. Because of great differences in carbohydrate density, the volume of a Zone Block of carbohydrate is highly variable. As an example, ¼ cup of cooked pasta and 3 cups of steamed broccoli both contain the same amount of carbohydrates (9 grams, or one Zone Block).

Of course, you don't want to forget fat. Guess how many blocks you need? That's right, three. Each fat block contains 3 grams of fat, so you'll get 9 grams of fat in three blocks and 12 grams in four blocks.

Another way to think of this is to use the "1-2-3" method. Plan to have 1 gram of fat for every 2 grams of protein and 3 grams of carbohydrate. A typical Zone meal for a woman would contain 10 grams of fat, 20 grams of protein, and 30 grams of carbohydrate.

However you do the calculations (the hand-eye, the Zone Block, or the "1-2-3" method), you will come up with virtually the same results. Whatever method you use, being in the Zone puts you in the driver's seat and literally takes away your enslavement to food. Remember, the Zone is not some mystical place but a state of hormonal balance that can only be achieved by the food you eat.

Before understanding the concept of the Zone, you may have seen yourself as a victim of the foods you crave. Maybe you've felt down and draggy and used some cookies or potato chips to give yourself energy and help you feel a little better. This measure only works temporarily, though, and you're soon left feeling even more tired after the short-term surge in energy wears off. You may feel like a strung-out addict looking for another fix. In a sense you are, but now you're looking for a fix of carbohydrates. This off-balance, out-of-control feeling is simply a consequence of your hormones being out of balance. The only way to break this habit is to get into the Zone.

You now have a pretty clear picture of what a typical Zone day is like. Knowing the rules of the Zone isn't enough, however. You need to be selective about the foods you choose. You need to aim for the highest-quality foods. You need to put the proper quality of fuel in your body to get the hormonal results you're looking for—whether you want to lose weight, live a healthier life, or reverse the course of a serious disease like Type 2 diabetes. Getting the right balance of carbohydrates, protein, and fat will only take you halfway there. Adding the highest-quality foods to this balance will take you the rest of the way.

chapter 3

The Healthiest Foods
in the World

You've no doubt heard that "you are what you eat." Considering what most Americans eat today, a lot of us are walking cheeseburgers and Twinkies. Unfortunately, the number of processed foods we have to choose from has increased exponentially due to advances in food technology combined with powerful marketing messages.

The good news is that you have more options than ever when it comes to healthful Zone food choices. If you choose wisely, you can make food your primary drug because of its power to alter your hormonal responses. The best food choices you can make are what I call the high-quality foods, the ones that generate the best hormonal responses in your body. *These high-quality foods will enhance the beneficial effects of the Zone.*

I devised a mathematical way of determining the quality of foods based on the effects that these foods have on all the systems in your body. Just like the octane rating of the gas you put into your car, the higher the quality of the food you use, the better the hormonal mileage. Combine high-quality foods with the Zone Diet, and you'll be maximizing the hormonal effects you get by being in the Zone.

In determining the foods that make my Top 100, I tapped into the USDA Nutrient Databases, which provide the vitamin, mineral, and nutrient content of nearly every food that's in the supermarket. You'll see that the mathematical equations are actually quite simple. And once you do the math, you'll be amazed by how many "nutritious" foods actually wind up being low in quality. In fact, many of the foods that the USDA recommends you eat daily in large quantities actually have little nutritional value—and wind up on my low-quality list.

HIGH-QUALITY CARBOHYDRATES: THINK ANTI-OXIDANTS

My definition of a high-quality carbohydrate is one that does two things: (1) provides anti-oxidants and (2) keeps your blood sugar and insulin levels as stable as possible. Anti-oxidants are essential because they quench free radicals, those unstable molecules in your body that wreak havoc on healthy cells and tissues. Excess free-radical production remains the biggest impediment to your quality of life. Although you need some free radicals to transform food into energy, any excess production of them (caused by eating too much food in general) triggers a breakdown in all areas of your body. Free radicals degrade your cellular DNA, which can turn a healthy cell into a cancerous one. They can also cause inflammation leading to heart disease, arthritis, and even wrinkles.

I firmly believe that within a few years the medical establishment will come to recognize that consistent inflammation in the body is the underlying cause of a great number of chronic disease conditions. Getting an abundant amount of anti-oxidants in your diet is one of your best biological defenses against disease and aging. The more anti-oxidant-rich foods you consume, the greater your ability to prevent free-radical-induced damage. What are the richest sources of anti-oxidants in your diet? Carbohydrates, in the form of fruits and vegetables.

It is well known that eating large amounts of fruits and vegetables is associated with lower levels of heart disease, cancer, and stroke. Since these are the three major causes of mortality in the Western world, it shouldn't be surprising that those populations who eat a lot of fruits and vegetables also live longer. While fruits and vegetables are rich in vitamin C and beta-carotene, new research is finding out that much of the anti-oxidative capacity of fruits and vegetables comes from other plant chemicals known as phytochemicals.

Plants have been conducting chemical warfare for billions of years and have developed a wide variety of anti-oxidative phytochemicals to protect themselves from their enemies. Only a few of these are termed *essential* anti-oxidants. This term is used to describe a true vitamin (like vitamins A, C, and E), which is a chemical that you must obtain through your diet. In fact, many of the so-called nonessential anti-oxidants are actually more powerful weapons against free radicals than the better-known vitamins. But you don't need to worry about whether your tomato has essential or nonessential anti-oxidants. Just follow this simple rule of thumb: The deeper the shade of purple in your plum or green in your lettuce, the more anti-oxidant power it has—which means it can quench more free radicals. The plant chemicals that bestow vibrant colors upon fruits and vegetables also contain their anti-oxidant powers.

To determine the top-quality carbohydrates for my Top 100 Zone Foods list, I considered three factors: anti-oxidative capacity, glycemic index, and soluble fiber content.

Factor #1: Anti-Oxidant Capacity

When calculating the highest-quality carbohydrates for my Top 100 list, I looked first at the fruit's or vegetable's total anti-oxidative capacity per gram of carbohydrate. This included not only the essential anti-oxidants such as vitamin A (often in the form of beta-carotene) and vitamin C, but also the broad array of nonessential anti-oxidants (like lycopene and other phytochemicals) that are packed into each gram of carbohydrate. Anti-oxidant capacity is based on the strength that a certain food has to neutralize a given number of free radicals. I ranked the fruits and vegetables based on their anti-oxidant capacity per gram of carbohydrate.

I use happy faces to rate the anti-oxidative capacity of a carbohydrate. The more happy faces, the greater the ability of a carbohydrate to fend off free radicals. The fewer free radicals your body has floating around, the happier and healthier you'll be. Here's a list of carbohydrates that have excellent anti-oxidative capacity (three happy faces), very good capacity (two happy faces), and a good capacity (one happy face).

Source	Anti-Oxidative Capacity (per gram of carbohydrate)
Excellent **(Zone Quality Greater Than 200)** ☺ ☺ ☺	
Vegetables	
Spinach	841
Kale	434
Romaine lettuce	387
Broccoli	254
Cauliflower	227
Fruits	
Blueberries	473
Blackberries	398
Strawberries	273
Very Good **(Zone Quality between 50 and 200)** ☺ ☺	
Vegetables	
Eggplant	159
Brussels sprouts	146
Red pepper	131
Cabbage	95
String beans	69
Onion	56
Fruits	
Plum	101
Pink grapefruit	63
Tomato	62
Kiwi	51

Good
(Zone Quality between 25 and 50)   ☺

Vegetables

Yellow squash	37
Celery	36
Cucumber	30

Fruits

Pear	44
Orange	42
Red grapes	42
Green grapes	30

What this type of ranking system allows you to do is compare one food with another in terms of anti-oxidative capacity per gram of carbohydrate. For example, on a gram-for-gram basis, blueberries (with a ranking of 473) have more than 10 times the anti-oxidative capacity of oranges (ranking of 42). Just glancing down the list, you'll quickly observe that the more colorful the carbohydrate, the greater its anti-oxidative potential.

Scientists haven't yet measured the anti-oxidative capacity of some foods. I calculated a rough estimate of the anti-oxidative capacity of each of these carbohydrates by measuring the amounts of vitamin C and A (as beta-carotene) contained in 9 grams of carbohydrate (one Zone Block of carbohydrate).

$$(\text{mg vitamin C}) \times (\text{mg beta-carotene})$$

Let's compare homemade cooked pasta and broccoli (one of the Top 100 Zone carbohydrates) using this equation.

Broccoli = (328 mg vitamin C) × (3.2 mg beta-carotene) = 1050

Homemade Pasta = (0 mg vitamin C) × (0 mg beta-carotene) = 0

Here's a list of low-quality carbohydrates, which have virtually no anti-oxidative capacity.

Exceptionally Useless Carbohydrates (Zone Quality of 0) ☹

- Bagels
- Pasta
- Rice
- Bread

What's astonishing is that these are the primary food items recommended in the U.S. government's dietary guidelines for Americans. I'm baffled by the fact that the government continues to push refined grain products even though these products are exceptionally dense in insulin-stimulating carbohydrates and have little anti-oxidative capacity. They simply have no redeeming features other than being cheap and plentiful.

To qualify for my Top 100 Zone Food list, a carbohydrate needs more than a strong anti-oxidative capacity. It must also pass muster on the glycemic index test.

Factor #2: Glycemic Index

This is a measure of how rapidly your body breaks down the carbohydrates in a particular food into the simple sugar glucose and how quickly this glucose gets into your bloodstream. The faster a carbohydrate gets into your bloodstream, the faster the rise in your blood sugar and the faster insulin is secreted to drive this excess glucose into storage sites in the muscles and liver.

The concept of the glycemic index only became well known during the past decade as nutritionists began to realize that many politically correct complex carbohydrates, like potatoes, actually caused faster rises in blood sugar than, well, table sugar. The more rapidly the blood sugar increases, the more insulin is released.

With all you know about Zone science, you can see why having a high-glycemic index is a no-no. The key to the Zone is keeping your insulin levels as stable as possible, which is why you want to consume foods with low glycemic indexes. (Actually, as I will show in Appendix B, the key is not just the glycemic index but the glycemic load, which takes into account the amount of carbohydrates a serving contains along with its glycemic index.) The Zone Diet has been criticized by nutritionists for excluding carrots, sweet potatoes, and corn. But these foods all have a relatively high glycemic index compared with other carbohydrates, which means they can cause dangerous rises in your insulin levels.

Factor #3: Soluble Fiber

This is the last factor I use to determine whether or not a carbohydrate is a top Zone food. Soluble fiber slows down the rate of entry of carbohydrates into the bloodstream, and this reduces insulin stimulation. This factor can move some of the relative losers on the anti-oxidative index into winners. This is the saving grace for apples, oatmeal, barley, and beans, which are relatively low in anti-oxidative capacity but high in soluble fiber.

To qualify for the Top 100 Zone Foods list, a carbohydrate should have at least 0.3 grams of soluble fiber per Zone Block of carbohydrate. Here are some examples of carbohydrates that do:

Carbohydrate	Grams Soluble Fiber per Zone Block
Kidney beans	0.5
Oatmeal	0.4
Apple	0.3

We're finally ready to determine whether a carbohydrate makes the cut for my list of Top 100 Zone Foods. In my Zone Food Quality Ranking System, I put together the three major factors (anti-oxidative capacity, soluble fiber, and glycemic index) in the following formula:

$$\frac{(\text{Anti-oxidative capacity per gram of carbohydrate}/100) \times (5 \times \text{Grams of soluble fiber per Zone Block})}{(100 - \text{Glycemic index})/100}$$

So let's revisit our previous example of broccoli versus homemade pasta. Broccoli, with an anti-oxidative capacity of 254, a soluble fiber content of 0.5 grams per Zone Block, and a glycemic index of 50 comes out like this:

$$\frac{[254/100] \times [5 \times (0.5)]}{(100 - 50)/100} = \frac{6.35}{0.5} = 12.7$$

Pasta, with an anti-oxidative capacity of 0, a soluble fiber content of 0, and a glycemic index of 59, comes out like this:

$$\frac{[0/100] \times [5 \times 0]}{(100 - 59)/100} = \frac{0}{0.41} = 0$$

You can see why broccoli is one of the top-ranked carbohydrates and gets three happy faces and why pasta is a very poor-quality carbohydrate that deserves its sad face ranking.

HIGH-QUALITY PROTEIN: THINK LOW FAT

I define the quality of a protein source by its fat content. Realize that all protein (even tofu) contains fat. *To qualify for my Top 100 Zone Foods list, a protein choice must contain at least twice as much protein as fat.* This eliminates most cuts of beef, pork, and lamb, with a few exceptions like well-trimmed beef tenderloin.

Switching from high-fat protein choices to lower-fat ones will reduce your intake of saturated fat. This will not only decrease cholesterol levels but also make the insulin receptors in your cells more responsive to insulin so that your body needs to make less of this hormone.

At the same time, you'll also slash your intake of health-damaging Omega-6 fatty acids, a type of polyunsaturated fat found in all sources of protein. This type of fat serves as the building block for certain types of eicosanoids that can accelerate the development of heart disease, cancer, Type 2 diabetes, and arthritis.

As with carbohydrates, I compare equal amounts of protein using the Zone Block method. This means that a smaller volume of lean protein will contain the same amount of protein as a larger volume of protein that is rich in fat (like a hot dog). So my formula for protein quality is the following:

Zone Block of protein/Total fat in that Zone Block of protein

For example, a skinless chicken breast that contains 7 grams of protein (one Zone Block of protein) also contains 0.4 grams of fat. Therefore its protein quality is

$$7 \div 0.4 = 18$$

Now let's compare a standard T-bone steak, which contains 7 grams of fat in one Zone Block of protein (7 grams of protein), and a skinless chicken breast.

T-Bone Steak = 7 grams protein ÷ 7 grams of fat = 1

This makes a chicken breast 18 times better than a T-bone steak as a Zone protein source.

I apply this formula to all types of protein—except fish. With fish, I factor in another fat that's exceptionally heart-healthy called long-chain Omega-3 fatty acids. These fats counteract the damage caused by excess Omega-6 fatty acids in your diet. Thus a fish protein choice can be higher in fat and still get a high rating, if the form of fat is long-chain Omega-3 fatty acids. Here is the revised equation for fish:

(Protein quality rating) + 50 × (Total long-chain Omega-3 fatty acids in one Zone Block of protein)

The higher the protein quality rating, the better the quality is for the preparation of Zone meals. Following are some of the Zone protein quality ratings.

Source	Zone Quality
Excellent Zone Protein	
(Zone Quality More Than 20) ☺ ☺ ☺	
Mackerel	44
Turkey breast	40
Haddock	30
Cod	30
Salmon	28

Soybean hamburger crumbles	25
Tuna steak	22
Turkey breast, deli	22
Lobster	21
Sea bass	20
Snapper	20

**Very Good Zone Protein
(Zone Quality Between 5 and 20)** ☺ ☺

Chicken breast	18
Freshwater bass	16
Trout	15
Cottage cheese (1%)	12
Chicken breast, deli	9
Tuna, canned in water	9
Soy imitation meat products	7
Emu	6

**Good Zone Protein
(Zone Quality Greater Than 2)** ☺

Pork tenderloin, well-trimmed	4
Tofu, extra-firm	4
Beef tenderloin, well-trimmed	3
Tofu, firm	3
Tempeh	2
Tofu, soft	2

Just as with carbohydrates, I consider more than one factor when ranking protein for its quality. Besides the fat content, I also look at the ability of a protein to regulate insulin levels. All protein raises insulin levels, although to a much lesser extent than carbohydrates. It turns out that soy protein has a much smaller effect on insulin than animal protein. For this reason I include many products containing soy protein on my Top 100

Zone Foods list, even though some products, like tofu, are relatively high in fat.

Examples of low-quality protein include the staples of most high-protein diets. These are fatty beef and pork products that contain relatively high amounts of fat and therefore high amounts of saturated and Omega-6 fats.

Low-Quality Protein
(Zone Protein Quality Less Than 1)   ☹

Ground beef (27% fat)	0.6
Sausage	0.3
Bacon	0.2

HIGH-QUALITY FAT: THINK MONOUNSATURATED FAT

Although I expend many more words discussing carbohydrates and protein, fat is not just a footnote. It's just as critical a part of the Zone. This is because high-quality fat will definitely fuel you better than low-quality fat. I define as high quality any food that's high in monounsaturated fats and low in saturated and Omega-6 fats. Saturated fat (found in whole milk dairy products and fatty red meat) can raise cholesterol levels, which leads to heart disease. Omega-6 fats, as mentioned above, can have adverse effects on the overproduction of "bad" eicosanoids associated with chronic disease. Monounsaturated fats, on the other hand, have no effect on insulin, cholesterol, or eicosanoids. Some research suggests that they may even raise "good" (high-density lipoprotein, or HDL) cholesterol levels. As a result, populations that consume high levels of monounsaturated fat have very low levels of cardiovascular disease and improved longevity.

My definition of high-quality fat is based on the fatty acid composition of one Zone Block of fat (3 grams of fat). The formula used to determine the quality of a fat is based on the relative amounts of these three types of fats within one Zone Block of fat, as shown below:

$$\frac{\text{(Grams of monounsaturated fat)}}{\text{(Grams of saturated fat)} + \text{(Grams of Omega-6 fat)}}$$

Here are some examples of high-quality and low-quality fats.

Source	Zone Quality
Excellent Quality Fats **(Zone Quality Greater Than 3)**	☺ ☺ ☺
Macadamia nuts	4.5
Olive oil	3.6
Olives	3.5
Very Good Quality Fats **(Zone Quality Between 2 and 3)**	☺ ☺
Avocado	2.3
Canola oil	2.2
Almond butter	2.2
Almonds	2.0
Good Quality Fats **(Zone Quality Between 1 and 2)**	☺
Cashews	1.6
Peanuts	1.1

Poor Quality Fats
(Zone Quality Less Than 1)   ☹
Lard	0.9
Butter	0.4
Safflower oil	0.2
Soybean oil	0.2

Macadamia nuts, which have a rating of about 4.5, contain the highest-quality fat you can find. Perhaps not surprisingly, macadamia nuts are also the most expensive nuts available. Olive oil is not far behind at 3.6. Research continues to confirm the health benefits of consuming more olive oil, to the point that it is now considered a heart-healthy idea.

Soybean oil (also known as vegetable oil) comes up with a measly rating of 0.2. This means that olive oil is 18 times better than soybean oil for making Zone meals. Ironically, soybean oil is the primary vegetable oil used in the United States. You may be amazed to discover that both lard and butter are lesser evils than vegetable oils. Although both are still poor-quality fats, they contain higher amounts of monounsaturated fat and lesser amounts of Omega-6 fatty acids.

One fat you should avoid at all costs is trans fatty acids, which are found in partially hydrogenated vegetable oils. Research has demonstrated that trans fatty acids are more damaging to your heart than saturated fats. Ironically, French fries used to be made with lard but are now made with "healthier" partially hydrogenated vegetable oils. Not only has the taste of French fries suffered as a result, but they now contain a far worse-quality fat that's more damaging to your arteries than lard.

PUTTING IT ALL TOGETHER

By now you should understand why combining a high-quality protein with a high-quality carbohydrate sprinkled with a dash of high-quality fat gives you a hormonally correct meal. In other words, the more happy faces you have with your ingredients, the happier your body will be and the happier you will feel. A great Zone meal is one that provides maximum insulin control for the next four to six hours. Consume one Zone meal after another, and you will achieve consistent hormonal control for your lifetime. Use low-quality foods, on the other hand, and you will simply lose the reins and allow your hormones to run wild. The choice should be easy to make.

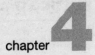

chapter 4

The Top 100 Zone Foods

You've seen the complicated equations that I use in my Zone Food Quality Ranking System. Now you can see how I put them to use to select foods for my Top 100 Zone Foods list. For each food, I provide a brief description of how the food benefits you, as well as an easy-to-follow recipe. (You can go to my web site, www.drsears.com, to view a photo of each prepared meal.)

The list is broken into four sections: carbohydrates, protein, fats, and spices and condiments. Within each section, the best-quality foods (three happy faces) are presented first, followed by the second-best (two happy faces), and concluding with the third-best (one happy face).

CARBOHYDRATES

Cauliflower ☺ ☺ ☺

Filling, high in fiber, and low in calories, cauliflower is a great food for reducing your waistline. Weighing in at only 25 calories, a cup of florets contains 100 percent of the recommended daily allowance (RDA) for vitamin C, one-third of the RDA for folate (although one-third of the folate is lost during cooking), and a nice serving of potassium and vitamin B_6. These nutrients all work to protect your heart. Folate and B_6, for example, both help break down homocysteine, a chemical that is known to cause artery damage. Cauliflower also contains bioflavonoids, indoles, and other chemicals that protect against cancer.

To retain the flavor of cauliflower and minimize nutrient loss, cook it rapidly by boiling or steaming. Overcooking cauliflower turns it mushy and releases sulfurous compounds, resulting in an unpleasant odor and bitter taste. When buying cauliflower, look for a head with firm, compact florets. Fresh cauliflower will have crisp green leaves and a snowy white head, or curd.

Did you know? *Cauliflower* literally means "cabbage flower." Centuries of agricultural advances were needed to produce a tight head of clustered flowered buds in place of the compact leaves on a cabbage head.

4 cups of cooked cauliflower = 1 Zone Block

Sicilian Cauliflower and Egg Frittata with Sausage and Peppers

Serves 1

Block size

½ Carbohydrate	2 cups cauliflower florets
1 Protein	1 whole egg
1½ Protein	3 egg whites
4 Fat	1⅓ teaspoons olive oil
1 Carbohydrate, 1½ Protein	1½ links "Lite Life" Italian tofu sausage
½ Carbohydrate	1 small onion, sliced
½ Carbohydrate	1 large green pepper, sliced
½ Carbohydrate	1 ripe tomato, sliced into wedges
1 Carbohydrate	1 cup strawberries, sliced

Cut off thick stem of cauliflower and discard. Separate cauliflower into florets by hand or with a knife. Chop remaining stalk or discard. Rinse and steam cauliflower in steamer basket over boiling water or in small amount of water with no basket until tender, about 10 minutes. Drain and mash gently with fork.

Beat egg and egg whites together. Put ⅔ teaspoon olive oil in a frying pan (nonstick, preferably) and heat on low. Add cauliflower evenly in pan and cook until lightly browned. Add eggs and cover. Keep flame as low as possible and cook frittata until almost done on top. Then loosen frittata around edges. Place serving dish large enough to cover frying pan over top. Flip frittata onto dish and immediately slip back into frying pan.

1

Cook 3 to 5 minutes longer until browned on second side. Set aside.

Break up sausage into bite-size pieces. Put ⅓ teaspoon olive oil in pan (cast iron, preferably) and spread with pastry brush. Add sausage and sauté on medium-high heat, stirring frequently until brown. Remove from pan.

Add remaining ⅓ teaspoon olive oil to same pan and sauté onion 3 to 5 minutes with 2 tablespoons water. Add green pepper and sauté 2 to 3 minutes, then add fresh tomato. There should be a little gravy. If not, add more water or broth, then cover and heat through for up to 5 minutes over low heat.

Serve frittata with sausage, pepper-and-onion mixture, and strawberries on the side.

Blackberries   ☺ ☺ ☺

Blackberries are loaded with vitamin C, fiber, and an assortment of phytochemicals that help protect against heart disease and cancer. Since they have among the highest anti-oxidative capacities of all carbohydrates, I call them nature's confections because they are still sweet enough to rival chocolate chip cookies or ice cream cake. Like apples, blackberries contain a huge dose of pectin, the type of fiber that mops up cholesterol by-products in the intestinal tract and carries them out of the body. This powerful fiber lowers circulating cholesterol levels without actually entering your bloodstream.

The vitamin C contained in berries helps protect blood vessels from the damaging effects of "bad" (LDL) cholesterol and also protects cells against damage by cancer-causing free radicals. A 1-cup serving has about 50 percent of the RDA for vitamin C. Adding to this nutritional arsenal is a wide variety of phytochemicals that have been shown to both inhibit cholesterol production and neutralize cancer cells. One particular phytochemical, ellagic acid, is a substance believed to help prevent cancer.

Although fresh blackberries are only in season during the summer months, you can get them all-year-round in the frozen version. Frozen blackberries will give you the same health benefits as the fresh kind, and you can use them anytime to sprinkle in green salads or mix into Zone smoothies.

Caveat: People who are allergic to aspirin may find that they experience a similar reaction from eating blackberries. This is because blackberries contain salicylate, an ingredient found in aspirin.

Did you know? There are several cultivated varieties of blackberries. Boysenberries are tart and dark maroon in color; loganberries are larger than wild blackberries, dark red, and very tart; and ollalieberries are shiny, black, and sweet.

¾ cup of blackberries = 1 Zone Block

Blackberry Custard Celebration

Serves 4

Block size

2 Protein	2 whole eggs
2 Protein and 2 Carbohydrate	2 cups 1% milk
	⅛ teaspoon vanilla extract (nonalcohol, glycerine base) or lemon zest
1 Carbohydrate	2 teaspoons sugar
1 Carbohydrate	⅔ cup blackberries

Beat eggs until they are light and fluffy. Then put eggs, milk, vanilla extract, and sugar in a nonstick saucepan. Heat mixture to a simmer, but not boiling. Pour mixture into four serving dishes and refrigerate to cool. After mixture has cooled for 20 minutes divide blackberries into the serving dishes and return to refrigerator. Serve when custard has set.

2

Blueberries   ☺ ☺ ☺

This is another extraordinary fruit that is high in anti-oxidative capacity. Like blackberries, blueberries are also rich in pectin, a soluble fiber that has been shown in several research studies to be effective in lowering cholesterol. At a mere 80 calories, a cup of blueberries provides nearly a third of the RDA for vitamin C and a considerable amount of potassium.

For centuries, dried blueberries have been a popular folk remedy for diarrhea and intestinal flu. Research has confirmed that blueberries can indeed combat "the runs" thanks to a substance contained in the berries called anthocyanin. This substance has mild antibiotic properties, especially against intestinal bacteria that cause diarrhea. The berries contain a substance that prevents bacteria from adhering to the bladder walls where they can multiply.

Interested in reversing aging? Blueberries may be able to help you along. The anti-oxidants in blueberries can help fight off free radicals from smog, cigarette smoke, and other offenders. One study from the National Institutes of Health found that rats that consumed blueberries were more active and more alert.

Did you know? Besides all their other health benefits, blueberries may be good for your eyes. A substance in blueberries called anthocyanin can help reduce eye-strain, according to a study from Japan.

½ cup of blueberries = 1 Zone Block

Blueberry Yogurt Breakfast

Serves 1

Block size

1 Protein	1 ounce lean Canadian bacon (substitute 3 turkey bacon strips or 2 soy sausage links)
1 Carbohydrate	½ cup fresh blueberries, rinsed and drained
3 Fat	1 tablespoon slivered almonds
2 Protein, 2 Carbohydrate	1 cup plain low-fat yogurt

Prepare bacon or soy links following package instructions. Stir fruit and nuts into yogurt, and serve with bacon or links on the side.

Broccoli   ☺ ☺ ☺

When President George Bush swore he would never eat broccoli, he probably didn't realize that he was forgoing one of the better nutritional bargains around. Over the past 20 years, numerous studies have concluded again and again that people who eat an abundance of broccoli have fewer cancers of the colon, breast, cervix, lungs, prostate, esophagus, larynx, and bladder. The reason lies in broccoli's abundance of disease-fighting compounds. For instance, broccoli contains indoles, compounds found in many cruciferous vegetables, which can help inactivate harmful estrogens that can promote the growth of tumors. Researchers at Johns Hopkins University discovered another compound in broccoli called sulforaphane that stimulates animal and human cells to produce cancer-fighting enzymes. As if this weren't enough, broccoli is also rich in beta-carotene, another well-known cancer fighter.

All in all, one broccoli spear contains about half the RDA for beta-carotene, more than twice the RDA for vitamin C, a healthy dose of potassium, and a decent amount of calcium, folic acid, and selenium. (Who needs a multivitamin?) And I wouldn't want to leave out the fact that broccoli packs a wallop of fiber. In fact, broccoli can be a great way to prevent constipation.

Did you know? Broccoli was rarely eaten in this country until 1923 when the D'Arrigo Brothers Company from Italy decided to do a trial planting of Italian sprouting broccoli in California. A few crates were sent to Boston, and by 1925 the nation was hooked on broccoli. Since then, our demand for broccoli has risen every year.

3 cups of cooked broccoli = 1 Zone Block

Broccoli-Ginger Chicken Delight

Serves 1

Block size

3 Fat	1 teaspoon olive oil
3 Protein	3 ounces boneless, skinless chicken breast, cut lengthwise into thin strips
½ Carbohydrate	1½ cups broccoli florets, washed
1 Carbohydrate	1½ cups snow peas, washed
½ Carbohydrate	¾ cup yellow onion, peeled and chopped
	1 teaspoon fresh ginger, grated
	¼ cup water
1 Carbohydrate	½ cup seedless grapes

In a wok or large nonstick pan, heat oil over medium-high heat. Add chicken and sauté, turning frequently, until lightly browned, about 5 minutes. Add broccoli, snow peas, onion, ginger, and water. Continue cooking, stirring often, until the chicken is done, water is reduced to a glaze, and vegetables are tender, about 20 minutes. If the pan dries out during cooking, add water in tablespoon increments to keep moist. Serve grapes for dessert.

Kale

☺ ☺ ☺

Kale may be one of those foods that you always hear is healthy, but you're not quite sure what to do with it once you have it in your refrigerator. That's a shame since it is one of the true superstars of the Top 100 list. The options are endless, and kale is definitely a carbohydrate that you don't want to skip.

A cup of kale has nearly 10,000 IU of vitamin A, almost twice the RDA. It has nearly a day's supply of vitamins C and E, two anti-oxidants that help ward off heart disease. Kale also contains some calcium, about 10 percent of the RDA in 1 cup. As if this weren't enough, kale is high in fiber and potassium. It's also rich in folate, the B vitamin that helps lower levels of the blood factor homocysteine that damages artery walls. Like other members of the cruciferous family, kale contains cancer-fighting compounds such as sulforaphane and indoles. Sulforaphane triggers the release of cancer-fighting enzymes, and indoles deactivate excess estrogens that can stimulate tumor growth.

Did you know? People have been eating kale for more than 4,000 years. The word *kale* was first used in Scotland and is derived from the Latin word *caulis,* meaning "cabbagelike plant." In fact, kale is one of the oldest members of the cabbage family.

2 cups of cooked kale = 1 Zone Block

Braised Lamb with Kale and Beans

Serves 1

Block size

4 Protein	4 ounces lean lamb, small dice
1 Carbohydrate	1½ cups onion, sliced
4 Fat	1⅓ teaspoons olive oil
	½ cup lemon-and-lime-flavored water
	½ teaspoon ground cinnamon
	⅛ teaspoon cayenne pepper
	Salt and pepper to taste
1 Carbohydrate	2 cups kale, torn
1 Carbohydrate	½ Granny Smith apple, roughly chopped
1 Carbohydrate	¼ cup white kidney beans

In a small pan sauté lamb and onion in hot oil until lightly browned. Add flavored water, cinnamon, cayenne, and salt and pepper. Cover, reduce heat, and simmer for 10 minutes. Add kale, apple, and beans. Bring to boil, reduce heat, cover, and simmer for 2 minutes to heat through. Place lamb on serving dish and arrange vegetables around it.

5

Lettuce
(Arugula, Butterhead, Romaine)   ☺ ☺ ☺

Not all lettuce is created equal. The color should clue you in. The deeper green the leaves, the more phytochemicals the lettuce contains—which is why the whitish, washed-out hue of iceberg lettuce just doesn't hack it compared with its more colorful cousins. Arugula, a member of the same plant family as broccoli, cabbage, and other cruciferous vegetables, is one of the most nutritious of all salad greens. A cup of arugula packs 2 mg of beta-carotene, 45 mg of vitamin C, 150 mg of calcium, and 0.5 mg of iron—all in just 12 calories.

Deeply colored lettuce greens are also rich in bioflavonoids, plant pigments known to work with vitamin C and other anti-oxidants to prevent cancer-causing cell damage.

Did you know? According to the writings of Herodotus, lettuce was served to the Persian kings as far back as the sixth century B.C. Lettuce was popular with the Romans at the beginning of the Christian era, and the Chinese grew lettuce beginning in the fifth century. The early colonists introduced lettuce to North America, and in 1806 sixteen varieties grew in American gardens.

10 cups of shredded lettuce = 1 Zone Block

Tomato Basil Salad

Serves 1

Block size

½ Carbohydrate	1 cup romaine lettuce, chopped
1 Carbohydrate	¼ cup chickpeas, rinsed and finely chopped
	1 tablespoon fresh parsley, chopped
4 Fat	1⅛ teaspoons olive oil
	1 tablespoon red wine vinegar
	2 tablespoons fresh basil, chopped
	1 teaspoon garlic, minced
	¼ teaspoon chili powder
2 Carbohydrate	4 tomatoes, sliced
4 Protein	4 ounces skim-milk mozzarella cheese, shredded

Place lettuce on a serving plate. In a medium bowl, combine chickpeas, parsley, oil, vinegar, basil, garlic, and chili powder. Alternate slices of tomato and shredded mozzarella on the lettuce bed. Pour chickpea dressing over tomatoes and serve.

Mustard Greens   ☺ ☺ ☺

If you've never tried mustard greens, you're in for a delicious treat. Young, tender leaves can be used in salads, while older leaves can be steamed for 15 to 20 minutes. Besides being flavorful, mustard greens give you a healthy dose of nutrients to combat cancer and heart disease. A cup of cooked mustard greens supplies nearly 100 percent of the RDA for beta-carotene and 50 percent of the RDA for vitamin C. Both of these anti-oxidants help protect against cancer and heart disease. They also give you more than 10 percent of a day's supply of iron and calcium. Iron protects against anemia, and calcium helps build strong bones and protects against osteoporosis.

Part of the cruciferous family, mustard greens will give you a shot of indoles, compounds that neutralize potent estrogens that stimulate the growth of tumors.

Did you know? Mustard plants are grown for their seeds in the western part of the United States. Indian mustards are grown for medical purposes and for their use in (yes!) mustard and other condiments. In Russia, mustard seed oil has been used as a substitute for olive oil.

4 cups of cooked mustard greens = 1 Zone Block

Tangier Chicken with Mustard Greens

Serves 2

Block size

8 Protein	1 pound chicken, skinless breast pieces with the bone (approximately half the weight of chicken breast is in bone)
	Salt and pepper to taste
8 Fat	2⅔ teaspoons olive oil
2 Carbohydrate	8 cups cooked mustard greens
	2 teaspoons cider vinegar
	3 cups chicken stock
1 Carbohydrate	1½ teaspoons honey
	⅛ teaspoon red wine
	¼ teaspoon gingerroot, grated
	½ teaspoon orange extract (nonalcohol, glycerine base)
1 Carbohydrate	4 teaspoons cornstarch
4 Carbohydrate	1⅓ cups mandarin orange sections

Preheat oven to 375°F. Sprinkle chicken with salt and pepper, then place in nonstick sauté pan with 2 teaspoons oil. Cook until browned. Then place chicken in baking dish and bake for 15 to 20 minutes. While the chicken is in the oven, place in the nonstick sauté pan used to brown the chicken the remaining ⅔ teaspoon of oil, mustard greens, and vinegar. Cook until mustard greens are almost tender. In small saucepan, blend

7

chicken stock, honey, wine, gingerroot, orange extract, and cornstarch. (Mix the cornstarch with a little water before adding it to the saucepan.) Heat mixture in saucepan, stirring occasionally until it is thickened. Remove chicken from oven and place chicken and orange sections in sauce. Do not allow orange sections to break up from overcooking. Simmer 3 to 5 minutes, then equally divide mustard greens on two dinner plates and top with an equally divided amount of chicken.

Raspberries   ☺ ☺ ☺

Nature's candy, the raspberry allows you to eat in the Zone without missing sugary tasting foods. Even better, a ½ cup serving contains 25 percent of the RDA for vitamin C, a decent amount of folate, potassium, and some iron. The potassium in raspberries can help prevent strokes and heart attacks by normalizing blood pressure. Vitamin C guards against cancer and cardiovascular disease and helps boost your immune system. Raspberries are extremely rich in anti-oxidative phytochemicals besides containing pectin, a soluble fiber that helps control blood cholesterol levels. The insoluble fiber in raspberries also helps promote bowel regularity. In addition, raspberries contain ellagic acid and other bioflavonoids that may help prevent some types of cancer.

Raspberries spoil faster than other berries because of their delicate structure and hollow core. Mold can grow quickly, so raspberries need to be consumed as quickly as possible after they are bought.

Did you know? The red raspberry was first cultivated about 400 years ago on European soil. In 1845 a physician in Philadelphia became the first successful producer of raspberries in this country, and he originated many varieties. By 1870 this berry had become an important crop in the United States.

1 cup of raspberries = 1 Zone Block

Raspberry Fruit Salad

Serves 4

Block size

4 Protein	1 cup low-fat cottage cheese
	Fresh ground black pepper to taste
1 Carbohydrate	⅛ cup mandarin orange sections*
1 Carbohydrate	½ apple, peeled, cored, and chopped
1 Carbohydrate	1 kiwi fruit, peeled and chopped*
1 Carbohydrate	1 cup raspberries*
4 Fat	4 crushed macadamia nuts
	Cinnamon

In a mixing bowl, combine cottage cheese and pepper, blend thoroughly, then place a quarter cup of peppered cottage cheese on each of four serving plates. In another mixing bowl, mix all fruits together to form a fruit salad. Place fruit salad around cottage cheese on the serving plates. Sprinkle with crushed macadamia nuts and cinnamon and serve.

Any other fruits in season can be substituted, as long as the Zone Blocks remain the same.

Spinach

☺ ☺ ☺

Popeye knew what he was doing when he downed his spinach. This green leafy vegetable packs a powerful nutritional punch, as it is the richest source of anti-oxidants per gram of carbohydrate. It is also rich in beta-carotene—1 cup of raw spinach has 3,690 IU of beta-carotene, or roughly 70 percent of the RDA. It also supplies two other carotenes, lutein and zeaxanthin, which protect your heart along with beta-carotene. Studies show that these carotenes keep circulating LDL, the "bad" cholesterol, from oxidizing, which can have damaging effects on your arteries. Spinach is also a good source of vitamin B_6, folic acid, iron, and potassium. It provides moderate amounts of riboflavin, vitamin C, calcium, and magnesium.

You can easily get the benefits from spinach year-round. Buy it in bunches in your produce section or in sealed bags that contain prewashed leaves. Use spinach in tossed salads as part of a mixture of greens or on its own.

Did you know? Adding a squirt of lemon juice to your spinach will not only give you extra flavor, but the vitamin C in lemon will help you absorb the iron in spinach.

3½ cups of cooked spinach = 1 Zone Block

Spinach Feta Pie

Serves 4

Block size

12 Fat	4 teaspoons olive oil
1 Carbohydrate	1½ cups large onion, chopped
2 Carbohydrate	4 medium red bell peppers, chopped
4 Fat	12 black olives, pitted and quartered
1 Carbohydrate	Six 10-ounce packages frozen chopped spinach, thawed and drained
	2 teaspoons garlic powder
	1 teaspoon sea or regular salt
1 Protein	1 large whole egg
15 Protein	15 ounces low-fat feta or soy cheese
4 Carbohydrate	1⅓ cups old-fashioned rolled oats
4 Carbohydrate	8 high-fiber crackers, such as Kavli or Wasa
4 Carbohydrate	1 medium cantaloupe, cut into 4 wedges or 2 grapefruits, quartered

Preheat oven to 350°F. In a large nonstick sauté pan, heat the oil over medium heat. Add the onion, red peppers, olives, spinach, garlic powder, and salt. Cook until heated through and most of the water is evaporated. In a large bowl, beat egg and crumble in feta. Add spinach mixture and set aside. To make crust, put rolled oats in blender or food processor with steel blade and pulse to create coarse oats. (Be careful not to overblend into a fine powder.) Add ⅓ cup of the ground oats to spinach mixture. Spread remaining oats into bottom of 9- by 13-inch Pyrex dish or large pie plate. Evenly distribute spinach and cheese mixture over oats. Bake for approximately 45 minutes or until pie is firm to the touch. Cut into 4 servings. Serve with crackers and fruit.

Strawberries   ☺ ☺ ☺

It may be hard to believe that a fruit as succulent as a strawberry is also a superstar when it comes to antioxidant power. In addition, 1 cup of strawberries gives you a whopping 140 percent of your RDA of vitamin C. Strawberries are also packed with flavonoids, two in particular, called quercetin and kaempferol. Research shows that these two flavonoids help keep "bad" (LDL) cholesterol from oxidizing and damaging artery walls.

As if this weren't enough, the strawberry contains ellagic acid, an amazing compound, also found in grapes and cherries, that has been shown to prevent carcinogens from turning healthy cells into cancerous ones. You can usually find strawberries year-round in the produce section, but their peak is usually spring through midsummer. Select strawberries that have a full red color, and avoid any that are uncolored or white. Make sure the berries on the bottom aren't mushy or moldy. Cut some strawberries into plain yogurt or blend into a soy smoothie.

Did you know? More than 70 varieties of strawberries are grown in the United States, and all are naturally sweet.

1 cup of strawberries = 1 Zone Block

Strawberry Mousse

Serves 6

Block size

3 Carbohydrate	3 cups fresh strawberries (the sweetest available)
3 Carbohydrate	2 tablespoons brown sugar
4 Protein	1 cup low-fat cottage cheese
1 Protein	4 tablespoons Just Whites* (mixed with water according to directions on the package)
1 Protein	1 envelope Knox Unflavored Gelatin, dissolved in purified water
6 Fat	6 teaspoons slivered almonds

Garnish (per serving):

1 Protein, 1 Carbohydrate	6 teaspoons plain low-fat yogurt
½ Carbohydrate	6 fresh strawberries (cut in a fan presentation)

Clean and core the strawberries, blend with the brown sugar, and let marinate for two hours. In a food processor fitted with a steel blade, puree the strawberries. Add the cottage cheese and puree again. Add the Just Whites and puree for uniformity. Finally add the dissolved gelatin, then pulse until thoroughly combined. Pour into

Just Whites are powdered egg whites.

10

six chilled wineglasses. Cover each with plastic wrap and refrigerate until the mousse is set. Top with the plain yogurt and strawberries and sprinkle almonds on top when ready to serve.

Swiss Chard   ☺ ☺ ☺

A member of the beet family, Swiss chard is another extraordinarily rich source of anti-oxidants. It also contains a great deal of vitamin C, beta-carotene, potassium, and calcium. Vitamin C is an anti-oxidant that can help prevent inflammation, which can lead to the aging of your skin, heart disease, and other chronic illness. Beta-carotene is another potent anti-oxidant that can have these same effects. You can eat the leaves, midsection, and roots of the Swiss chard. You can throw it into salads or in a stir-fry with other vegetables. Don't overcook Swiss chard, however, because its vitamin content decreases through cooking.

Swiss chard is great when combined with other vegetables in a salad, and it may even help ward off colds. Swiss chard can also benefit your digestive system because it contains many of the vitamins and minerals that promote proper digestive function. It's amazingly low in calories for all the health benefits it confers.

Did you know? Chard was the beet of the ancients. Aristotle wrote about red chard, and Theophrastus mentioned light-green and dark-green chard in the fourth century B.C. Chard was used as a potherb in the Mediterranean, Asia Minor, and the Middle East long before Roman times.

2½ cups of cooked Swiss chard = 1 Zone Block

Salade Montreux

Serves 1

Block size

4 Fat	1⅓ teaspoons olive oil, divided
4 Protein	4 ounces Canadian bacon, diced
	2 teaspoons balsamic vinegar
	½ teaspoon Dijon mustard
	Salt and pepper to taste
1 Carbohydrate	½ cup Zoned Herb Dressing (see page 68)
½ Carbohydrate	6¼ cups Swiss chard, raw
1 Carbohydrate	2 cups canned mushrooms, sliced
½ Carbohydrate	1 cup scallions, sliced (white and green parts)
1 Carbohydrate	½ Granny Smith apple, cored and chopped

In a nonstick sauté pan, heat ⅓ teaspoon oil. Lightly brown the Canadian bacon in the oil. Blend 1 teaspoon oil, balsamic vinegar, mustard, and salt and pepper into the Zoned Herb Dressing. Combine Swiss chard, mushrooms, scallions, apple, and bacon in serving bowl. Add dressing, toss to coat, and serve.

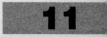

11

Zoned Herb Dressing

Four ½-cup servings

Block size

1 Carbohydrate	1½ cups onion, finely minced
1 Carbohydrate	¼ cup chickpeas, canned, finely minced
2 Carbohydrate	8 teaspoons cornstarch
	1¾ cups purified water
	¼ cup cider vinegar
	2 tablespoons balsamic vinegar
	⅛ teaspoon Worcestershire sauce
	1 teaspoon dried tarragon
	1 teaspoon dried oregano
	1 teaspoon parsley flakes
	2 teaspoons garlic, minced
	1 teaspoon dried basil
	⅛ teaspoon chili powder
	½ teaspoon celery salt
	1 teaspoon dried dill

Combine all ingredients in a small saucepan to form a thickened dressing. (Mix cornstarch with a little cold water to dissolve it before adding to saucepan.) Heat dressing to a simmer, constantly stirring until mixture thickens. Transfer dressing mixture to a storage container, let cool, and refrigerate. Each time you make a Zone-favorable meal, use this dressing as a replacement for 1 Carbohydrate Zone Block.

Kohlrabi   ☺ ☺ ☺

A cross between a turnip and a cabbage, kohlrabi can be steamed and served hot with a Zone protein choice or cooked and sliced cold for salads. The cruciferous vegetable is very rich in vitamin C—1 cup contains 150 percent of the RDA. It also contains a hefty dose of potassium and more than 10 percent of the RDA for vitamin E.

Kohlrabi has an unusual appearance that sets it apart from other members of the cabbage family. Instead of a head of closely packed leaves, it has a long oblong-shaped stem and leaves like a turnip. The most popular varieties in the United States are White and Purple Vienna.

When choosing kohlrabi, select bulbs that are young since they don't need to be peeled like older bulbs, which are very tough. The bulb is the only edible part of the plant, even though the leaves contain more nutrients.

Did you know? *Kohlrabi,* a German word that means "cabbage turnip," made its way across Europe during the sixteenth century. It was brought to America during the early 1800s.

1 cup of cooked kohlrabi = 1 Zone Block

Kohlrabi Curry

Serves 1

Block size

4 Fat	1⅛ teaspoons olive oil
	1 teaspoon cumin seed
	1 teaspoon mustard seed
	1 large clove garlic, minced
	1 to 2 inches fresh gingerroot, peeled and grated to equal 1 tablespoon
	Pinch of freshly ground black pepper
	1 tablespoon curry powder (preferably Madras/hot)
4 Protein	8 ounces extra-firm tofu, cut into cubes
2 Carbohydrate	2 cups cooked kohlrabi
2 Carbohydrate	3 cups fresh green beans, cut into 1-inch pieces
	¼ cup vegetable stock (see page 71)

Heat oil in large sauté pan over medium heat. Add cumin and mustard seed and cook until coated. Add minced garlic, grated ginger, black pepper, and curry powder. Sauté for 1 minute to blend flavors. Add tofu, kohlrabi, beans, and vegetable stock. Cook, stirring occasionally, for 10 to 15 minutes or until kohlrabi is tender. Serve immediately.

12

Vegetable Stock

Approximately 6½ cups stock

Block size

2 Carbohydrate	2 cups leeks
2 Carbohydrate	2 cups carrots, chopped
1 Carbohydrate	1½ cups onion, coarsely chopped
1 Carbohydrate	2 cups celery, coarsely chopped
¾ Carbohydrate	1 large zucchini, chopped
	1 bunch fresh parsley
	½ bunch fresh thyme
	7 whole peppercorns
	8 cups purified water

Trim leeks by cutting away dark green ends and bulb. Cut in half and wash thoroughly. Coarsely chop. Put all ingredients into a large stockpot. Bring to a boil, then simmer 1½ to 2 hours. Strain through a fine sieve or strainer. Cool. Refrigerate or freeze and use as necessary.

Turnip Greens   ☺ ☺ ☺

If you eat turnips and discard the greens, you don't know what you're missing. From a nutritional standpoint, the greens are a far better choice than the turnip itself. A cup of boiled greens provides 40 mg of vitamin C (two-thirds of the RDA), about 200 mg of calcium, and nearly 300 mg of potassium. This compares with the turnip's 18 mg of vitamin C, a measly 35 mg of calcium, and 210 mg of potassium. What's more, turnip greens yield nearly 4,000 IU of vitamin A (in the form of beta-carotene), which is 80 percent of the RDA. As a member of the cruciferous family (along with broccoli and cabbage), turnips contain sulfurous compounds that may protect against certain forms of cancer.

Caveat: Turnip greens may cause bloating and gas when you first start eating them. Eat them boiled, baked, steamed, or braised rather than raw to limit gas, and eat small amounts at first.

Did you know? Some practitioners of herbal medicine recommend turnips, either fresh, as a juice, as a syrup, or as a pack placed over the chest, to treat bronchitis and sore throats. This remedy hasn't been proven in research studies.

4 cups of cooked turnip greens = 1 Zone Block

Fertile Crescent Greens

Serves 1

Block size

½ Carbohydrate	¾ cup onion, minced
4 Fat	1⅓ teaspoons olive oil
	1 clove garlic, pressed
	2 tablespoons fresh coriander (1 tablespoon if dried)
	¼ teaspoon crushed hot red pepper
	½ teaspoon salt
	¼ teaspoon allspice
1 Carbohydrate	1 cup shelled fresh or frozen broad beans
3 Protein	1 cup soy hamburger crumbles
	1½ cups vegetable stock (see page 71)
½ Carbohydrate	2½ cups turnip greens, washed and chopped fine
½ Carbohydrate	Juice of ½ lemon
½ Carbohydrate	1 medium tomato, chopped
1 Protein	1 soy sausage patty
1 Carbohydrate	1 plum

Sauté onion in oil 5 to 7 minutes in skillet over medium-high heat. Add garlic, coriander, hot red pepper, salt, and allspice. Stir 1 to 2 minutes. Add beans and soy crumbles and stir another 2 to 3 minutes until coated and warm. Add vegetable stock. Cover and simmer on low heat until beans are tender, 25 to 30 minutes with

13

fresh beans. (Cooking time with frozen beans will vary. See package.) Just as the beans are finishing, add the turnip greens, stir well, cover, and steam 5 to 7 minutes. Serve piping hot topped with lemon juice and chopped tomato, and a heated sausage patty on the side. Serve plum for dessert.

Apricots   ☺   ☺

Nobel Prize winner G. S. Whipple in 1934 touted apricots as "equal to liver in hemoglobin regeneration." Fresh apricots are rich in iron and vitamin C, an antioxidant that helps your body absorb iron—hence the explanation behind Whipple's quote. Much of the vitamin C is lost, however, when apricots are dried or canned.

Apricots are most well known for their ability to help prevent certain cancers, specifically cancers of the lung and pancreas. The reason? Apricots contain extremely concentrated amounts of beta-carotene, a form of vitamin A that has been shown to prevent the division and growth of cancer cells in cell culture. Laetrile, a controversial remedy derived from apricot pits, was hailed as a new cure for cancer during the 1970s but has since been found to be ineffective. In fact, laetrile has been banned in this country because apricot pits and other sources of laetrile contain cyanide, which can be toxic if consumed in large amounts.

Caveat: Sulfite preservatives in some dried apricots can trigger an allergic reaction or asthma attack in people susceptible to these disorders. In addition, a natural salicylate in apricots may trigger an allergic reaction in aspirin-sensitive people.

Did you know? When King Solomon said, "Comfort me with apples for I am sick," he was really talking about apricots. Eve reached for an apricot in the Garden of Eden—not an apple. And the apricot is cherished in the

Himalayan kingdom of Hunza (the land of Shangri-La in the novel *Lost Horizon*) as a source of health and exceptional longevity.

3 apricots = 1 Zone Block

Creamy Apricot Crunch

Serves 4

Block size

1 Carbohydrate	⅛ cup rolled oats cooked
1 Fat	3 cashews, chopped
1 Fat	1 macadamia nut, chopped
2 Fat	6 almonds, chopped
2 Carbohydrate	4 teaspoons pure maple syrup, divided
4 Protein	4 ounces skim ricotta cheese
	½ tablespoon pure vanilla extract (nonalcohol, glycerine base)
	½ tablespoon orange extract (nonalcohol, glycerine base)
	1 teaspoon cinnamon
1 Carbohydrate	3 medium apricots, sliced

In a dry skillet, gently roast oats, cashews, macadamia nut, and almonds over medium heat. Stir to keep from burning. Mix in 2 teaspoons maple syrup and remove from heat. In a separate bowl, beat ricotta vigorously with vanilla and orange extracts, cinnamon, and remaining 2 teaspoons maple syrup. Mixture will start out curdlike. Beat by hand or with mixer until smooth and creamy. Spoon ricotta onto each of four chilled plates and top with apricot slices and oat-nut crunch.

14

Artichokes   ☺ ☺

Contrary to its name, the Jerusalem artichoke is not a true artichoke but a member of the sunflower family. The true artichokes are the cone-shaped cardoon and the globe. The globe is the more popular of the two. Some people complain that artichokes require too much effort to eat, but I love scraping the flesh off the leaves with my teeth and savor the reward of the fleshy heart in the center. Diving into a freshly steamed artichoke is a culinary adventure!

A large artichoke provides 15 percent of the RDA for folate and vitamin C, 300 mg of potassium, about 2 grams of fiber, and is plentiful in calcium and iron as well. A series of studies in 1940 by a Japanese researcher found that the artichoke lowered total cholesterol somewhat, stimulated production of bile in the liver, worked as a diuretic, and enhanced "well-being strikingly." Follow-up studies confirmed the artichoke's cholesterol-lowering effects. These beneficial effects may come from a chemical in artichokes called cynarin. In fact, cynarin was formulated into a drug for lowering blood cholesterol.

When choosing artichokes, select those that are compact, plump, and heavy and yield slightly to pressure. Their leaves should be large and tightly clinging and a nice green color. An artichoke is overripe when its leaves are spreading and the center is fuzzy or dark pink or purple.

Did you know? The name *artichoke* is derived from the northern Italian words *articiocco* and *articoclos*, which refer to a pinecone. (Makes sense, since the artichoke does resemble a pinecone.) Artichokes were brought to England from the Mediterranean in 1548, and French settlers planted them in Louisiana in the mid–nineteenth century. California now produces the largest artichoke crop in this country, with its peak season in March, April, and May.

4 artichokes or 1 cup of artichoke hearts = 1 Zone Block

Artichoke and Mushroom Ragout

Serves 1

Block size

4 Fat	1⅓ teaspoons canola oil
1 Carbohydrate	4 cups mushrooms, sliced, raw
	½ cup vegetable stock (see page 71)
2 Carbohydrate	3 cups canned peeled tomatoes, chopped
1 Carbohydrate	1 cup canned artichoke hearts, chopped
	½ teaspoon oregano, dried and ground
	¼ teaspoon thyme, dried and ground
	Salt and pepper to taste
	1 tablespoon parsley, minced
4 Protein	8 ounces extra-firm tofu, cut into 1-inch slices

Heat oil in a heavy, nonreactive saucepan over high heat. Sauté mushrooms 4 minutes or until lightly browned. Add stock and boil until mixture is reduced by half. Add tomatoes, artichoke hearts, oregano, thyme, and salt and pepper to taste. Simmer 4 minutes, stirring frequently, until sauce thickens. Stir in parsley and remove from heat. Set aside and keep warm. Turn on broiler. Season tofu with pepper to taste. Arrange tofu on a broiler pan and broil 3 to 4 minutes per side or until golden. Serve tofu topped with sauce.

15

Asparagus   ☺   ☺

Asparagus root contains compounds called steroidal
glycosides, which may help reduce inflammation. In
fact, some Chinese herbalists have used it to treat arthritis. Western medicine doesn't recognize the healing
powers of asparagus, but the vegetable does contain
healthy doses of anti-oxidants. Just ½ cup of cooked asparagus provides about 25 percent of the RDA for folic
acid and more than 80 percent of the RDA for vitamin
C. Asparagus is also a fair source of potassium, fiber,
and beta-carotene.

The rich trove of vitamins, minerals, and phytochemicals in asparagus may help protect against cervical cancer, colon and rectal cancer, and heart disease. It
can also help protect your immune system. What's
more, the folic acid it contains may help to prevent birth
defects. Asparagus acts like a natural diuretic to help
prevent water retention.

Caveat: Asparagus needs to be cooked as soon as possible after buying. It can lose half its vitamin C and much
of its flavor if it's left unrefrigerated for two or three
days. Store it refrigerated, wrapped in a damp cloth or
waxed paper until it is ready to be eaten.

Did you know? The ancient Greeks and Romans
thought that asparagus possessed medicinal qualities,
curing everything from rheumatism to toothaches.
None of these claims have proven true.

12 asparagus spears = 1 Zone Block

Asparagus Tofu Dip

Serves 4

Block size

½ Carbohydrate, 4 Protein	12 ounces of regular tofu (not extra-firm)
	1½ tablespoons umeboshi vinegar (Japanese plum vinegar; *not* the same as regular vinegar—umeboshi is salty and tangy)
	1 tablespoon brown rice vinegar or fresh lemon juice
	1½ tablespoons Dijon or stone ground mustard
	Optional: 2 scallions, trimmed and minced
4 Fat	1⅓ teaspoons olive oil, or 12 black olives, chopped
	2 to 4 tablespoons + 3 cups purified water
	½ teaspoon sea salt
1 Carbohydrate	12 asparagus spears
½ Carbohydrate	2 cups cauliflower, cut into bite-size florets
1 Carbohydrate	1 large daikon (Japanese white radish), cut into sticks
1 Carbohydrate	2 red or orange bell pepper, seeded, cut into long strips

16

Boil or steam tofu for 4 minutes, then drain. Crumble tofu into a blender or food processor. Add vinegar, mustard, (optional) scallions and olive oil or olives. Blend until smooth and creamy. Add water a tablespoon or two at a time as needed to create a smooth texture like sour cream. Pour into four custard cups, cover, and chill for at least 3 hours to allow flavors to meld.

Meanwhile, bring 3 cups salted water to a boil in an uncovered 2-quart saucepan. Cook each type of vegetable separately but in the same boiling water, until crisp but tender. Cook about 2 to 4 minutes: more for asparagus and cauliflower, less for bell peppers. Remove vegetables with a large skimmer basket and transfer to a colander. Run vegetables under cold water to stop the cooking and hold the color.

Place each dish of tofu dip on a large dinner plate. Arrange vegetables in concentric circles or mounds around the dish. Serve cold.

Bok Choy

☺   ☺

Also called Chinese mustard cabbage, bok choy resembles a cross between celery and green Swiss chard. It is, in fact, a member of the cabbage family, but bok choy is no ordinary cabbage. It is far and away the healthiest type of cabbage you can eat. A cup of chopped bok choy contains nearly the entire RDA for beta-carotene, but that's not all. Bok choy is also rich in vitamin C, potassium, and calcium. A cup of bok choy has roughly the same amount of calcium as ½ cup of milk.

Like other cruciferous vegetables, bok choy packs a powerful disease-fighting punch with indoles, phytochemicals that are believed to deactivate potent estrogens that can stimulate the growth of tumors, particularly in the breast. Researchers from the National Cancer Institute are investigating these health benefits and should know more in the next few years.

Although the raw leaves of bok choy have a slightly sharp tang, cooking turns the leaves milder and the stalks sweeter.

Did you know? Bok choy can make the perfect cold remedy. Sprinkle ½ cup raw bok choy in a bowl of hot chicken soup. The antibiotic effects from the chicken soup combined with the anti-oxidants in bok choy will help you fight off nasty cold and flu viruses.

3 cups of cooked bok choy = 1 Zone Block

Vietnamese Spring Lettuce Rolls with Peanut Dressing

Serves 1

Block size	
4 Protein	8 ounces extra-firm tofu, cubed
1 Carbohydrate	½ cup carrots, grated
⅓ Carbohydrate	1 cup bean sprouts, washed and dried
⅓ Carbohydrate	2 stalks bok choy, washed and shredded
¼ Carbohydrate	½ small sweet onion, such as Walla Walla or Vidalia, grated
½ Carbohydrate	¾ cucumber, peeled and grated
¼ Carbohydrate	½ red bell pepper, cut in ¼-inch strips
¼ Carbohydrate	½ yellow bell pepper, cut in ¼-inch strips
	1 tablespoon fresh mint, finely chopped
3 Fat	1 teaspoon peanut oil
	2 teaspoons lime juice
	1 teaspoon rice wine vinegar
	1 to 2 inches gingerroot, peeled and grated to equal 2 teaspoons
	1 tablespoon chives, chopped
	¼ teaspoon salt, or to taste
	6 large red leaf or green leaf lettuce leaves, washed and patted dry

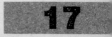

| 1 Fat | 6 peanuts, finely chopped |
| 1 Carbohydrate | 1 kiwi for dessert |

In a medium-size bowl, combine tofu, carrots, bean sprouts, bok choy, onion, cucumber, red and yellow pepper, and fresh mint. Set aside. In a jar with a lid, put peanut oil, lime juice, rice wine vinegar, ginger, chives, and salt. Close lid and shake dressing until well mixed. Taste and adjust seasoning. Coat tofu and vegetables with dressing and toss together. Spoon equal amounts of mixture onto lettuce leaves, sprinkle with peanuts, and roll up. Serve chilled.

Barley   ☺ ☺

Barley is one of only two grains (the other is oatmeal) on the Top 100 Zone Foods list. Although barley is carbohydrate-dense like other grains, it is unique because it is rich in soluble fiber that helps prevent spikes in your blood sugar levels—which is a major problem with other grains.

Barley is an excellent source of soluble fiber and has been shown to lower blood cholesterol levels. A noteworthy Australian study of 21 men with mildly high cholesterol levels showed that when they were given a diet rich in barley products, their cholesterol levels dropped an average of 6 percent overall. What's more, "bad" LDL cholesterol declined by 7 percent. A similar report from Montana State University found even better results: people on a high-barley diet experienced a 12 percent drop in total cholesterol. Barley appears to work by interfering with the liver's manufacture of cholesterol, probably by the reduction of insulin levels.

Did you know? For about 6,000 years barley has been hailed as a food that makes you potent and vigorous. Roman gladiators, called *hordearii* ("barley eaters"), consumed the grain to store up energy. In Pakistan, some refer to barley as "medicine for the heart."

½ **tablespoon of dry barley = 1 Zone Block**

Barley-Mushroom Soup with Smoked Tofu

Serves 1

Block size

2 Carbohydrate	1 tablespoon barley
	4 cups vegetable stock (see page 71)
4 Fat	1⅓ teaspoons olive oil
½ Carbohydrate	¾ cup onion, chopped
¼ Carbohydrate	2 medium stalks celery, chopped
¼ Carbohydrate	8 medium mushrooms, sliced
½ Carbohydrate	¼ cup tomato puree
4 Protein	8 ounces smoked (or plain) extra-firm tofu, cubed
	1 medium sprig parsley, minced
½ Carbohydrate	1 medium ripe tomato, chopped
	Salt and pepper to taste
	Optional: vegetarian Worcestershire sauce, (available at health food stores)

Combine barley and vegetable stock in medium stock-pot, bring to a boil, and simmer for 20 minutes. In a separate pan, sauté olive oil, onion, and celery over medium-high heat for 4 to 5 minutes. Add mushrooms, increase heat to high, and brown for 3 to 4 minutes, until mushrooms release their juice. Add sauté and

18

tomato puree to barley broth. Simmer for 20 minutes. Add cubed tofu and simmer 5 minutes longer. Serve in hefty bowls, topped with parsley, fresh tomato, salt, pepper, and vegetarian Worcestershire sauce.

Bell Peppers, Red   ☺ ☺

Red peppers add zest and beauty to all kinds of green salads. You may not know that red peppers are really just a more mature form of green peppers, which were allowed to ripen longer on the vine. (Depending on their ripeness, bell peppers range in color from green to yellow to red.) For this reason, red peppers are packed with the most plentiful amount of nutrients. Still, both kinds of peppers are rich in vitamin C; one pepper provides about 150 percent of the RDA for vitamin C—about the same as an orange or grapefruit.

Red peppers are one of the few foods that contain lycopene, a phytochemical that may help prevent various forms of cancer. Some research has found that people with low levels of lycopene have a greater risk of developing cancers of the cervix, bladder, and pancreas. As if this weren't enough, the average red pepper has 4,220 IU of beta-carotene, more than 80 percent of the RDA for this vitamin. (Green peppers have about half that amount.) This is why red peppers have a greater anti-oxidative capacity than green peppers.

Did you know? Peppers were named by Spanish explorers, who confused them with the unrelated peppercorn.

2 red peppers = 1 Zone Block

Bell Pepper Stir-Fry

Serves 1

Block size

4 Fat	1⅓ teaspoons olive oil, divided
4 Protein	8 ounces extra-firm tofu, diced
	⅛ teaspoon celery salt
	½ teaspoon Worcestershire sauce
1 Carbohydrate	2 cups red and yellow bell peppers, chopped
½ Carbohydrate	¾ cup onion, chopped
1 Carbohydrate	¼ cup chickpeas, rinsed
	1 teaspoon garlic, minced
	1 tablespoon cider vinegar
	Dash of hot pepper sauce
	⅛ teaspoon paprika
1 Carbohydrate	2 tomatoes, chopped
	⅓ cup lemon-and-lime-flavored purified water
½ Carbohydrate	2 teaspoons cornstarch
	Dash of lemon herb seasoning

In a medium-size nonstick sauté pan, heat ⅔ teaspoon of oil. Add tofu, celery salt, and Worcestershire sauce, and stir-fry until browned and crusted on all sides. In a second pan, heat remaining oil. Add peppers, onion, chickpeas, garlic, vinegar, hot pepper sauce, and paprika. Cook until the vegetables are tender. Add tomatoes,

19

water, and cornstarch. (Mix cornstarch with water to dissolve it before adding to sauté pan.) Combine tofu and vegetable mixture. Spoon onto serving plate and sprinkle with lemon herb seasoning.

Black Beans   ☺ ☺

Black beans are amazing regulators of insulin. Yes, they are carbohydrate-dense, but the massive amounts of soluble fiber they contain help slow the entry of glucose into the bloodstream. This means that you produce much less insulin in response to eating beans compared with other lower-quality carbohydrates.

Black beans are native to South America and are used throughout the area as a staple to be boiled, fried, spiced, and mixed with rice and other foods. Black beans are traditionally made into black bean soup in Cuba, Puerto Rico, and Spain.

Caveat: Don't go overboard on beans if you're not used to having them in your diet. Gradually add them to your diet by starting with ¼ cup of cooked beans one to two times a week. Your body will soon adjust to the increased fiber intake. Also, drink extra water to help your gastrointestinal tract handle the extra fiber. Realize that the more processed the bean is, the more rapidly it enters the bloodstream. As an example, black bean soup has a glycemic index nearly double that of boiled black beans.

Did you know? Beans were eaten often by the ancient Greeks, who would hold a "bean feast" to honor Apollo. Although beans were once called "poor man's meat," they have come into their own thanks to Americans' renewed interest in nutritious, high-fiber foods.

¼ cup of cooked black beans = 1 Zone Block

Black Bean Salsa

Serves 4

Block size

3 Carbohydrate	¾ cup canned black beans, drained and rinsed
1 Carbohydrate	2 tomatoes, diced
¼ Carbohydrate	½ small red onion, chopped
4 Fat	1⅓ teaspoons olive oil
	Juice of 1 lime
	4 tablespoons cilantro, chopped
	½ jalapeño pepper, or to taste
	Pinch of salt, or to taste
	Pinch of freshly ground pepper, or to taste
4 Protein	4 ounces of low-fat cheddar cheese

Mix black beans, tomato, red onion, olive oil, lime juice, and cilantro in a medium-size bowl. Seed jalapeño pepper by cutting in half and taking out seeds. Since the heat of the pepper is mostly in the seeds, you may want to wear rubber gloves or be careful working with pepper. Finely chop half the pepper and add to mixture. Add salt and pepper. Taste and adjust seasoning. For more "heat," cut remaining jalapeño pepper and add to salsa. Sprinkle cheese on top.

Cabbage ☺ ☺

If you consider yourself a savvy shopper, cabbage is one of the best nutritional bargains around. Both red and green cabbages are among the least expensive and most disease-protective foods you can buy. A cup of shredded cabbage gives you almost 70 percent of your vitamin C needs and a good dose of potassium to help fight high blood pressure. Green cabbage, more so than red, will meet 10 percent of your daily folate requirement. This B vitamin helps fend off heart disease by clearing the artery-damaging chemical homocysteine from the circulation. What's more, cabbage has a high content of cholesterol-clearing soluble fiber. Who could ask for a better bargain?

Caveat: Cabbage stinks, literally, when it's cooked. The more you cook it, the more it releases its foul-smelling sulfurlike compounds. Flash-cook cabbage by quickly stir-frying or lightly steaming it.

Did you know? Cabbage appears to be the mother of all cruciferous vegetables. There is evidence that cabbage was grown more than 4,000 years ago, and those centuries of cultivation have produced other forms of the cabbage family, which include kale, kohlrabi, cauliflower, broccoli, and (you guessed it!) brussels sprouts.

3 cups of cooked cabbage = 1 Zone Block

Stuffed Cabbage

Serves 1

Block size

	5 medium-size cabbage leaves, rinsed
3 Fat	1 teaspoon olive oil
½ Carbohydrate	¾ cup medium onion, minced
1 Fat	3 black olives, pitted and finely chopped
½ Carbohydrate	½ tablespoon raisins, finely chopped
	¼ teaspoon paprika
	¼ teaspoon garlic powder, or 1 clove garlic, minced
	¼ teaspoon sea or regular salt
	⅛ teaspoon black pepper
4 Protein	8 ounces extra-firm tofu, drained and crumbled
1 Carbohydrate	½ cup tomato sauce
2 Carbohydrate	⅔ cup unsweetened applesauce

In a covered glass bowl, microwave cabbage leaves in 1 tablespoon water for 4 minutes or until desired texture. Set aside to cool. Heat oil in sauté pan over medium heat. Sauté onion, olives, and raisins for approximately 5 minutes or until onion turns translucent. Add paprika, garlic, salt, and pepper. Cook another 2 minutes. Add tofu and 2 tablespoons of tomato sauce. Cook another 5 minutes. Wrap filling in cabbage leaves. Serve with remaining tomato sauce. Serve applesauce for dessert.

21

Eggplant   ☺   ☺

Eggplant's deep purple hue is an obvious tip-off that this vegetable packs a powerful wallop of free-radical-fighting phytochemicals. Phytochemicals not only give fruits and vegetables their brilliant colors but also are potent cancer and heart disease fighters because of their ability to quench free radicals before they do any significant damage. In addition, nasunin, which gives eggplants their purple color, has been shown to help lower blood cholesterol levels. Eggplants also contain terpenes, phytochemicals that may deactivate steroidal hormones that can promote the growth of certain types of tumors and may also protect against oxidative damage that can make a cell susceptible to cancerous growth.

Eggplant is also good for your heart. It gives you a moderate dose of potassium, which helps stabilize blood pressure, and is very low in fat and calories—unless, of course, you bread it and deep-fry it.

Did you know? Eggplants bear no relationship to eggs—nor does the shiny purple vegetable resemble an egg. So how did it get its name? Turns out that a very early variety of eggplant, grown hundreds of years ago, was small, white, and shaped like an egg, hence the name.

1½ cups of cooked eggplant = 1 Zone Block

Tofu-Eggplant Gumbo

Serves 1

Block size

4 Fat	1⅓ teaspoons olive oil, divided
4 Protein	8 ounces extra-firm tofu
	Celery salt, to taste
1 Carbohydrate	1½ cups onion, chopped
½ Carbohydrate	1 cup green bell pepper, chopped
½ Carbohydrate	1 cup celery, sliced
1 Carbohydrate	2 tomatoes, crushed
1 Carbohydrate	1½ cups eggplant, peeled and diced
	2 cups vegetable stock (see page 71) or bouillon
	2 teaspoons garlic, chopped
	½ teaspoon dried thyme
	⅛ teaspoon cayenne pepper
	¼ cup fresh parsley, chopped
	Optional: salt and pepper to taste

In a medium-size nonstick sauté pan, heat ⅔ teaspoon oil. Add tofu and sprinkle with celery salt. Stir-fry over medium-high heat until browned and crusted on all sides, about 5 minutes. Transfer browned tofu to a platter, lightly cover with aluminum foil to keep warm, and set aside. Heat remaining oil in a 10- to 12-inch skillet. Add onion, bell pepper, celery, tomato, and eggplant. Add stock, garlic, and remaining spices except the salt and pepper and bring to a boil. Reduce heat and cook, covered, stirring occasionally until vegetables are almost tender, about 10 minutes. Add salt and pepper to taste. Remove cover and continue cooking over high heat until liquid thickens and vegetables are tender, about 5 minutes more. Spoon gumbo into a shallow soup bowl and top with tofu.

Fennel   ☺ ☺

With a fat white bulb and green stalks, fennel may look like celery, but it has its own health benefits and distinct licorice flavor. Although it is from the same family as celery, fennel is even more nutritious. A 1-cup serving fulfills one-third of the RDA for vitamins A and C. It also provides 15 percent of the RDAs for iron and calcium, as well as potassium and other minerals.

You can eat all parts of the fennel plant, and you can prepare and serve it in many ways. It can be raw in salads or braised, steamed, baked, or sautéed as a side dish. Stuffed and baked fennel bulbs are a great vegetarian main course, and the chopped leaves can be used as a garnish for vegetable soups.

Did you know? Fennel has been in the medicine bags of physicians through the ages. Hippocrates recommended fennel tea to stimulate milk production in nursing mothers. Ayurvedic physicians in India have long prescribed fennel seeds to aid digestion and prevent bad breath. Fennel may even have been the first diet drug. Ancient Greek and Roman healers used fennel seeds to prevent obesity, and modern herbalists recommend fennel tea as a diet aid.

¾ cup of raw fennel = 1 Zone Block

Citrus-Tofu Fennel Salad

Serves 1

Block size

2 Carbohydrate	1½ cups fennel bulb
2 Carbohydrate	1 orange
4 Protein	8 ounces extra-firm tofu,
	patted dry and diced
	2 sprigs watercress, chopped
4 Fat	1⅓ teaspoons olive oil
	Juice of ½ lime
	Pinch of salt, or to taste

Cut fennel bulb in half, then thinly slice. Blanch fennel in boiling water. Remove and dunk into ice bath to cool. Drain. Peel orange, and section by cutting away thin membrane around segments. Retain juices and pulp in small bowl. Set aside. In medium-size bowl, mix together tofu, fennel, orange segments, and watercress. Set aside. To orange juice and pulp, add olive oil, lime juice, and salt. Toss tofu, fennel, and orange with dressing. Arrange on plate and serve.

Grapefruit   ☺ ☺

Every diet plan seems to begin the day with half a grape-fruit, which contains just 40 calories. (There's even a diet with just grapefruit!) But grapefruit confers so many more health benefits than simply its low-calorie status. Grapefruit packs in lots of nutritional goodies, supplying a heaping dose of vitamin C, folic acid, and potassium—all of which protect your heart. Pink grape-fruit is relatively rich in anti-oxidants, and ruby red grapefruit provides an added bonus: lycopene, the phy-tochemical that helps prevent the "bad" (LDL) choles-terol from oxidizing and damaging artery walls. As if this weren't enough, grapefruit also contains pectin, a soluble fiber that reduces the rate of entry of carbohy-drates into your bloodstream, thereby lowering insulin secretion.

Grapefruit and other citrus fruits also protect against cancer. In Japanese studies, grapefruit extract stopped tumor growth after it was injected under the skin of mice. The researchers concluded that grapefruit is a "remarkable anti-mutagen," a substance that re-verses cellular changes that lead to the division and growth of cancer cells.

To maximize the heart benefits, be sure to eat the grapefruit pulp, which includes the membranes that sep-arate the sections and the white interior of the rind. These are the areas that contain pectin, and that's why grapefruit juice (which has none of this pulp) is not high in pectin and doesn't lower cholesterol levels.

Did you know? In 310 B.C., the Greek historian Theophrastus wrote of grapefruit: "A decoction of the pulp of this fruit is thought to be an antidote to poison, and will also sweeten the breath." Later Pliny, the Roman naturalist who first used the word *citrus*, labeled the fruit a medicine.

½ grapefruit = 1 Zone Block

Grapefruit Winter Fruit Compote

Serves 1

Block size

3 Protein	¾ cup low-fat cottage cheese
	⅛ teaspoon cinnamon
	⅛ teaspoon nutmeg
1 Carbohydrate	½ grapefruit, in sections
1 Carbohydrate	⅓ cup mandarin orange sections
3 Fat	3 teaspoons almonds, slivered and toasted
1 Carbohydrate	½ Granny Smith apple, cored and chopped
	Paprika

In a small mixing bowl, combine cottage cheese with cinnamon and nutmeg. Mound onto serving dish. Arrange grapefruit and orange sections around cheese. Combine almonds and apple pieces, and spoon onto cheese. Sprinkle paprika over cheese and serve.

24

Green Beans   ☺ ☺

Although technically a legume, green beans are more like vegetables than beans. Green beans don't pack in as many carbohydrates or calories as other beans, so you can eat them in larger quantities on the Zone Diet. Green beans are rich in vitamins A and C, two powerful anti-oxidants that can help protect your arteries from damage by free radicals. They also contain some calcium and phosphorus.

When choosing green beans, select ones that are crisp and tender and without scars. They should snap readily when broken. Those with well-shaped pods and small seeds are usually the best tasting. The beans should feel pliable and velvety. To enhance their nutritional value, flavor green beans with oregano, basil, or dill.

Did you know? Green beans are native to South America and were introduced into Europe in the sixteenth century. Over 150 varieties of green and yellow snap beans are grown today.

1½ cups of cooked green beans = 1 Zone Block

Poached Haddock with Hot Green Beans and Artichokes

Serves 4

Block size

	1 cup purified water
	½ cup onion, sliced thin
	2 cups 2% milk
	¼ teaspoon sea salt
	Pepper
12 Protein	4 haddock fillets, each weighing 5 ounces for a total of approximately 20 ounces
	Parsley to garnish

Sauce:

3 Fat	1 teaspoon butter
	1½ tablespoons flour
	1 cup poaching liquid
	Optional: 20 green grapes

Marinade:

	3 tablespoons lemon juice
	⅓ cup red wine vinegar
	¼ cup olive oil

| 11 Carbohydrate | 4 quarts of french cut green beans |
| 1 Carbohydrate | 1 cup drained artichoke hearts |

25

9 Fat

1 tablespoon olive oil
½ cup chopped parsley
¼ cup chopped chives
Optional: 2 tablespoons
chopped pimiento

In a large skillet, preferably stainless steel or enameled cast iron, bring the water and onion to a boil. Add the milk, salt, and pepper, then add the fish fillets. Reduce the heat and cook for 5 or 6 minutes. Turn off the heat and remove the fillets to a warm platter.

Over medium heat, reduce the poaching liquid by half. Meanwhile, prepare the sauce. In a small saucepan, over medium heat, melt the butter. Add the flour and cook for a minute, while whisking, to cook the flour. Whisk in half the cup of poaching liquid. The sauce will thicken immediately. Add the rest of the liquid and whisk well. Add green grapes and return the sauce to a boil. Adjust the seasoning and serve the sauce with Hot Green Beans and Artichokes over the fish and garnish with parsley.

Mix marinade ingredients together. Toss green beans and artichoke hearts in marinade. Keep in a covered glass dish in the refrigerator until ready to cook.

Drain off as much of the marinade as possible. Heat the olive oil in a large skillet. Toss beans and artichoke hearts until heated through (about 3 or 4 minutes). Add parsley and chives. You can add chopped pimiento for color at the last minute.

Brussels Sprouts   ☺ ☺

Although high on the "yeech" factor, brussels sprouts can actually be a delicacy—if you prepare them right. They also rank high on my list of the Top 100 Zone Foods, so you should consider developing a taste for them. Looking like tiny heads of cabbage, brussels sprouts are indeed a member of the cabbage family and confer many of the same health benefits as other cruciferous vegetables. Brussels sprouts are packed with indoles and sulforaphane, two powerful phytochemicals that can neutralize cancer cells. The vegetable also contains important vitamins and minerals and assorted other anti-oxidative phytochemicals. A 1-cup serving contains a fair amount of beta-carotene and potassium, 150 percent of the RDA for vitamin C, and more than 10 percent of the RDA for iron and vitamin E.

Caveat: Brussels sprouts often produce gas, but steaming or boiling them over low heat can help you avoid trouble. If you do experience gas, start with a ½-cup serving of the sprouts until your body gets used to them.

Did you know? As the name suggests, brussels sprouts are said to be native to Brussels, Belgium. English farmers began growing them early in the nineteenth century, but no one thought to grow them here until early in the twentieth century.

1½ cups of cooked brussels sprouts = 1 Zone Block

Mustard-Glazed Brussels Sprouts with Tofu

Serves 1

Block size

4 Fat	1⅓ teaspoons olive oil, divided
	½ teaspoon Worcestershire sauce
	⅛ teaspoon celery salt
4 Protein	8 ounces extra-firm tofu, ½-inch dice
2 Carbohydrate	3 cups brussels sprouts, frozen
	1 teaspoon garlic, minced
1 Carbohydrate	½ cup Zoned Tarragon Mustard Sauce (see page 110)
1 Carbohydrate	1½ cups red onion, chopped
	Salt and pepper to taste

Heat ⅔ teaspoon oil in a medium-size nonstick sauté pan. Blend in Worcestershire sauce, celery salt, and tofu. Stir-fry until browned and crusted on all sides. In a medium saucepan, cook brussels sprouts according to package directions. Remove from pan and drain. In a second nonstick sauté pan, heat remaining oil and garlic. Stir in sprouts, Zoned Tarragon Mustard Sauce, and onion. Stir-fry until onion is tender. Place sprout mixture on serving plate and top with tofu. Salt and pepper to taste.

26

Zoned Tarragon Mustard Sauce

Four ½-cup servings

Block size

2 Carbohydrate	½ cup chickpeas, canned, finely minced
2 Carbohydrate	8 teaspoons cornstarch
	2 cups chicken stock
	2 tablespoons cider vinegar
	½ teaspoon Worcestershire sauce
	2 teaspoons dried tarragon
	2 teaspoons ground mustard
	¼ teaspoon turmeric
	2 teaspoons garlic, minced

Combine all ingredients in a small saucepan. (Mix cornstarch with a little cold water to dissolve it before adding to saucepan.) Heat sauce to a simmer, constantly stirring with a whip until mixture thickens. Transfer sauce mixture to a storage container, let cool, and refrigerate. This sauce may be refrigerated for up to 5 days or, if you prefer, frozen and defrosted for later use. Although the sauce is freeze-thaw stable, after it has been frozen and defrosted it may need to be stirred to reincorporate the small amount of moisture that forms on it during the freezing and thawing process.

Kiwi ☺ ☺

You probably think of it as an exotic fruit, and indeed, kiwi is native to New Zealand, but you should make this fruit less foreign to your refrigerator because it is bursting with vitamin C. One kiwi has 120 percent of the RDA for this disease-protective vitamin. Besides helping to boost your immune system, vitamin C is an anti-oxidant that can protect your arteries from the damaging effects of free radicals. Kiwi is also rich in potassium, which can help maintain the proper fluid balance in your body's cells while helping to maintain normal heart function and blood pressure.

Kiwis can be picked while green and can be kept in cold storage for 6 to 12 months, which makes them available for most of the year. Ripe kiwis can be eaten raw. You can even eat the skin if it is defuzzed. An enzyme (actiniolin) found in kiwi can be used as a natural meat tenderizer. Rub the meat with a cut kiwi 30 to 60 minutes before cooking to tenderize tough meat without imparting any flavor from the fruit.

Did you know? The kiwi originated in China and was known as the Chinese gooseberry until New Zealand fruit growers renamed it for their national bird and began exporting it. Now grown in California, kiwis have become increasingly plentiful in supermarkets.

1 kiwi = 1 Zone Block

Kiwi Fruit Salad with Walnuts

Serves 4

Block size

4 Protein	4 envelopes Knox Unflavored Gelatin
	2 cups purified water
1 Carbohydrate	1 kiwi fruit, peeled and diced
1 Carbohydrate	1 cup raspberries*
1 Carbohydrate	1 cup strawberries, diced*
1 Carbohydrate	½ cup seedless red grapes, halved
4 Fat	4 teaspoons walnuts, chopped
	1 tablespoon banana extract (nonalcohol, glycerine base)
	1 tablespoon orange extract (nonalcohol, glycerine base)
	½ teaspoon strawberry extract (nonalcohol, glycerine base)
	Mint leaves

Place gelatin and water in a saucepan, and stir until dissolved, then add fruits, nuts, and extracts. Heat to a simmer, stirring gently for 10 minutes until the raspberries dissolve. Pour liquid into an 8-inch-square 2-inch-deep pan and let cool. When set, place in four serving dishes and garnish with mint leaves.

When choosing berries, look for those that are medium-size and uniform in color. They should also feel solid to the touch and not be leaking juice.

Lentils   ☺   ☺

Like other legumes, lentils have a healthy dose of soluble fiber, which helps regulate blood sugar levels; this improves insulin and reduces your risk of diabetes. Soluble fiber has also been shown to reduce cholesterol levels, which can reduce your risk of heart disease. Lentils contain a fair amount of protein, although they are primarily carbohydrates and are low in fat and calories. They pack a hefty amount of nutrients: extremely rich in folic acid, they also contain respectable levels of potassium, iron, and copper.

Did you know? In the Bible, Esau sold his birthright to his brother Jacob for a bowl of lentil soup. With all of lentils' health benefits, he might not have gotten such a bad bargain after all.

¼ cup of cooked lentils = 1 Zone Block

Savory Lentils with Goat Cheese

Serves 1

Block size

4 Carbohydrate	1 cup lentils, rinsed and drained
	½ teaspoon salt, divided
	2 cups purified water
	1 clove garlic, minced
	2 tablespoons cilantro
	2 tablespoons chives, chopped
4 Fat	1⅓ teaspoons olive oil
	Juice of 1 lime
4 Protein	4 ounces goat cheese, room temperature
	⅛ teaspoon freshly ground pepper, or to taste
	2 radicchio leaves for garnish

In a medium-size saucepan, place lentils, ¼ teaspoon of the salt, and water. Bring to a boil and simmer for about 20 minutes or until lentils are tender but still have texture. Remove from heat and drain. In a medium-size bowl, mix lentils, garlic, cilantro, and chives together. Add olive oil and lime juice. Toss gently. Before serving, fold in goat cheese. Season with remaining salt and pepper. Arrange radicchio leaves on plate. Spoon salad onto radicchio. Serve chilled, at room temperature, or warm.

28

Nectarines   ☺ ☺

Sweeter and more nutritious than its cousin the peach, the nectarine is especially high in beta-carotene, an anti-oxidant that your body converts to vitamin A. One medium-size fruit supplies 20 percent of the RDA for vitamin A. It's also high in potassium, giving you 150 mg, and rich in vitamin C, supplying 7 mg or 10 percent of the RDA.

The yellow flesh of nectarines is rich in bioflavonoids, especially carotenoids. These plant pigments are anti-oxidants that protect your heart from the damaging effects of free radicals. They also reduce your risk of developing cancer. As if all these nutrients weren't enough, nectarines are also high in pectin, a soluble fiber that helps control cholesterol levels.

Did you know? Nectarines were named after the Greek god Nekter. Their juice was later called the drink of the gods. There is no basis to the myth that a nectarine is a cross between a peach and a plum; it actually began as a genetic variant of the peach.

½ nectarine = 1 Zone Block

Nectarine Yogurt Freeze

Serves 8

Block size

4 Protein, 4 Carbohydrate	2 cups plain low-fat yogurt
3 Protein	3 envelopes Knox Unflavored Gelatin
3 Carbohydrate	1½ medium nectarines, halved, pitted, and chopped
1 Carbohydrate	2 teaspoons sugar
	⅛ teaspoon ginger
	Dash of allspice
	2 teaspoons vanilla extract (nonalcohol, glycerine base)
1 Protein	2 egg whites
8 Fat	8 teaspoons slivered almonds, chopped

In saucepan, place yogurt, gelatin, fruit, sugar, spices, and extract. Heat until mixture becomes thoroughly warm, no more than 180°F. Cool and set aside. In a mixing bowl, whip egg whites until firm. When the mixture in the saucepan has cooled, combine it with the whipped egg whites and chopped almonds. Pour mixture into a pan and place in freezer, or add mixture to an ice-cream maker and blend. When mixture is frozen, scoop into eight small serving dishes.

29

Oats (Slow-Cooked)   ☺ ☺

Long before cholesterol became a sworn enemy, Americans began the day with a warm bowl of oatmeal. In the 1950s, oatmeal was replaced with higher-fat fare like bacon and eggs and French toast. Oats made a comeback in the 1980s, when cholesterol became a notorious bad guy that we needed to attack with a vengeance. Oats, it turns out, have a special fiber called beta-glucan that acts like a sponge in your intestines, mopping up cholesterol and bile (made from cholesterol) and then exiting with the bound bile in your stool. Studies show that just a serving a day of oats can improve your cholesterol levels.

Slow-cooked steel-cut oats are the most nutritious kind of oats and should really be the only kind you choose on the Zone plan. Processed oats found in breakfast cereals and instant oatmeal can cause spikes in your blood sugar and insulin levels comparable to the effects of white flour. Slow-cooked oatmeal is digested more slowly because it contains more soluble fiber. Thus you get more gradual rises in blood sugar, which keeps you in the Zone.

Did you know? Oat bran has done lots of nutritional flip-flops: First it was hailed as a cure-all for high cholesterol levels in the 1980s. Then it was panned by a 1990 research study that found it was no more effective than white bread in lowering cholesterol. Recent studies have vindicated oat bran (contained primarily in slow-cooked oatmeal) as a cholesterol-lowering agent. Researchers now think that eating 3 grams of oat bran a day can lower cholesterol levels by 5 to 6 points—

which can reduce your heart disease risk by as much as 12 percent.

⅓ cup of cooked oatmeal = 1 Zone Block

Grandma's Oatmeal

Serves 1

Block size

3 Carbohydrate	1 cup cooked oatmeal
3 Protein	21 grams of protein powder
3 Fat	3 teaspoons slivered almonds

Add 3 cups of salted water to ⅓ cup of the oatmeal. Bring to a boil, let simmer for 30 minutes. Add the protein powder after cooking the oatmeal to fortify it.

30

Okra ☺ ☺

This low-calorie vegetable is high in folate, with a ½-cup serving containing 50 percent of the RDA. It is also a rich source of the anti-oxidant vitamins A and C and of potassium. The biggest bonus offered by okra is its high fiber content. One of these fibers, pectin, helps lower blood cholesterol levels by interfering with bile absorption in the digestive tract and forcing your liver to take cholesterol from the blood to make bile. Other soluble fiber in okra helps stabilize blood sugar levels, preventing dangerous spikes in insulin levels.

Some people find that okra, with its gummy consistency, is an acquired taste. To enhance the taste, cook okra with an acidic vegetable like tomatoes to reduce its gumminess; also try steaming or blanching it rather than boiling it to keep the vegetable crisper.

Did you know? If you love Cajun cooking, you've probably eaten okra—maybe without even knowing it. Okra is used by southern cooks to thicken a Cajun stew called gumbo. In fact, okra is nicknamed gumbo in many parts of the world.

1 cup of cooked okra = 1 Zone Block

Shrimp Gumbo

Serves 1

Block size

4 Fat	1⅓ teaspoons olive oil
½ Carbohydrate	1 cup celery, sliced
1 Carbohydrate	1½ cups onion, chopped
1 Carbohydrate	1½ cups tomatoes, chopped
½ Carbohydrate	½ cup frozen okra, sliced
1 Carbohydrate	¼ cup frozen corn kernels
	½ teaspoon hot pepper sauce (or to taste)
	½ teaspoon garlic, minced
	¼ teaspoon chili powder
	⅛ teaspoon celery seed
4 Protein	6 ounces small shrimp, shelled and deveined
	¼ teaspoon paprika
	½ teaspoon lemon herb seasoning
	⅓ cup lemon-and-lime-flavored water

Heat oil in a medium-size nonstick sauté pan. Add the celery, onion, tomatoes, okra, corn, hot pepper sauce, garlic, chili powder, and celery seed. Cook until vegetables are tender. Mix in the shrimp, paprika, lemon herb seasoning, and flavored water. Simmer 3 to 5 minutes until the shrimp are cooked. Spoon into a medium bowl and serve.

31

Oranges   ☺ ☺

Packed with 130 percent of your daily vitamin C needs, more than 20 percent of the fiber, and 12 percent of the folate as well as a good dose of potassium, an orange comes with a powerful disease-fighting arsenal. The vitamin C can lower your cholesterol levels and protect your artery walls from damage that can lead to plaque buildup. A host of research studies have also found that the fiber in oranges, pectin, can help bring high cholesterol levels down to the safe zone.

The orange is also a potent weapon against cancer. Vitamin C can counteract powerful cancer-causing substances called nitrosamines. In one study, those who ate the most oranges had about half the cancer risk of those who ate the least. Scientists have also studied oranges for their ability to combat viruses. Investigators found in one research study that oranges helped to lessen the respiratory symptoms caused by the rubella virus.

Did you know? Spanish explorers brought oranges to Florida during the time of Ponce de Leon's quest for the Fountain of Youth. Orange seedlings were cultivated at the San Diego Mission, California, in 1769, and by the year 1804, 400 seedlings had grown into a grove. The popularity of the orange increased until it became known as "California's liquid sunshine."

½ orange = 1 Zone Block

Orange, Tofu, and Spinach Salad

Serves 4

Block size

¼ Carbohydrate	1-pound package prewashed baby spinach or flat leaf spinach, stemmed, washed, spun dry, torn into large pieces
¼ Carbohydrate	½ grated carrot
½ Carbohydrate	½ Walla Walla Sweet or Vidalia onion, cut into thin rings
2 Carbohydrate	1 seedless orange, peeled and sectioned, or ⅔ cup mandarin orange sections
1 Carbohydrate	⅓ cup water chestnuts, drained
4 Protein	4½ to 6 ounces smoked tofu, cubed
	1-inch piece of fresh gingerroot
	½ tablespoon umeboshi plum vinegar (*not* the same as regular vinegar—umeboshi is salty and tangy)
	1 tablespoon purified water
4 Fat	1⅓ teaspoons untoasted sesame or almond oil

Place spinach in a large serving bowl. Top with grated carrot, onion rings, orange sections, water chestnuts, and tofu cubes. Wash gingerroot and peel with paring knife or vegetable peeler. Grate on the smallest hole of a standard grater or use special ginger grater. Grab pulp, make fist, and squeeze over a small bowl or tablespoon. Wet pulp with a few drops of water, squeeze again, then discard pulp. Combine ginger juice, umeboshi plum vinegar, water, and oil. Whisk with a fork. Pour over salad and toss until salad wilts slightly. Transfer to a large salad plate and serve.

Variation

Replace tofu with 1 hard-boiled egg or 2 hard-boiled egg whites and 3 ounces of cubed skim or part skim cheddar, Colby, or other cheese. Prepare as previously instructed.

Plums ☺ ☺

The plum is now one of the most popular fruits in the world, second only to the apple. No doubt plums are chosen for their great taste, but they also contain a host of nutrients and significantly high anti-oxidative capacity. One medium-size plum contains only 36 calories and is a good source of fiber, including pectin, which can help lower cholesterol levels. It also provides vitamin C, riboflavin, and potassium. A plum also promotes regularity—in fact, a prune is a dried plum.

Fresh plums don't ripen after they have been picked, so buy ones that are brightly colored and yield slightly to your touch. I recommend against picking canned plums over fresh ones since they contain only one-sixth the amount of vitamin C. (This nutrient is lost when plums are skinned and heated during canning.)

Did you know? The plum tree plays a significant role in Chinese mythology and is associated with great age and wisdom. Blossoms of the plum tree are carved on jade to signify resurrection.

1 plum = 1 Zone Block

Plum Cheese Supreme

Serves 1

Block size

	¼ to ⅛ cup purified water (less for a gas range; more for electric)
	¼ teaspoon powdered anise or whole anise seeds
1 Carbohydrate	1 tablespoon raisins or currants or 2 dates, minced
3 Carbohydrate	3 plums, peeled if waxed, seeded, halved, and cut into thin wedges
4 Protein	4 ounces low-fat mozzarella, Colby, Monterey Jack, or cheddar-style soy cheese, grated or cut in thin strips
4 Fat	12 lightly toasted almonds or 4 macadamia nuts, coarsely chopped

Add water, anise, raisins, and plum to an 8- or 9-inch skillet with a lid. If cooking for two, use two small skillets or one 10- to 12-inch skillet. Cover and bring to boil. Reduce heat and simmer for about 4 to 6 minutes or until almost tender. While fruit cooks, grate cheese. Remove lid from skillet; sprinkle nuts, then cheese over fruit. Cover and simmer for 2 to 3 minutes or until cheese melts. (Or simply cover, remove from heat, and let stand 3 to 4 minutes until cheese melts.) Remove

33

from heat. Use a spatula to slide the dish onto a dinner plate. Serve immediately.

Variation

Replace the 12 almonds or 4 macadamia nuts with 12 toasted pecan halves. Prepare as previously instructed.

Radishes   ☺ ☺

A member of the cruciferous family, the radish is a cousin of cabbage, kale, turnips, and cauliflower and shares many of the same health benefits. A radish provides some vitamin C and small amounts of iron, potassium, and folate. It also provides sulfurous compounds that may protect against cancer.

When selecting radishes, choose those with a bright color, which indicates freshness. The vegetables should feel solid and have an unblemished surface. Remove any leaves and tops; the radishes will stay fresh longer without the tops.

You can grow radishes fairly easily in a backyard garden. They can grow in all types of soil, although they may require plant food. Some varieties mature in just twenty-one days, but the winter variety takes about sixty days. You can cook the roots and tops and/or use them raw in salads.

Did you know? Even before the Egyptian pyramids were built, ancient records indicate that radishes were a common food in that country. An ancient Greek physician wrote an entire book on radishes.

4 cups of radishes = 1 Zone Block

Spicy Tofu with Scallions and Radishes

Serves 1

Block size

4 Fat	1⅓ teaspoons olive oil
	1 teaspoon gingerroot, minced, divided
4 Protein	8 ounces extra-firm tofu, 1-inch cubes
	1 tablespoon lemon juice
	1 tablespoon purified water
	4 teaspoons soy sauce
	½ tablespoon white wine
	1 teaspoon garlic, minced
	Salt and pepper to taste
1 Carbohydrate	1½ cups jalapeño and red bell pepper, finely diced (mixed to desired heat)
½ Carbohydrate	10 cups fresh spinach, torn
¼ Carbohydrate	1 cup radishes, thinly sliced
1 Carbohydrate	1½ cups tomatoes, seeded and diced
½ Carbohydrate	½ cup scallions, chopped
¾ Carbohydrate	1½ cups canned mushrooms, sliced

Heat oil and ½ teaspoon gingerroot in medium-size sauté pan. Stir-fry tofu until browned on all sides. Add spinach and cook until wilted. Whisk lemon juice,

34

water, soy sauce, wine, garlic, salt and pepper, and remaining gingerroot together in a small bowl. Combine vegetables in a medium bowl and pour in soy sauce mixture. Toss to coat. Add in tofu and spoon onto serving dish.

Tomatoes   ☺ ☺

Eating a tomato a day may actually keep the cancer doctor away. Tomatoes contain a unique carotenoid called lycopene. Research suggests that people who have the highest blood levels of lycopene may be at a much lower risk of developing various forms of cancer, including cancers of the cervix, bladder, and pancreas. Just eating one tomato a day can give you this protective effect. Even better news: you don't need to eat a raw tomato. Lycopene is present in processed tomato products such as tomato juice and tomato paste. Tomatoes are also an excellent source of vitamin C and have some fiber.

Did you know? Brought to Europe from Central America by the Spanish during the sixteenth century, tomatoes were grown as decorative plants and often referred to as poisonous love apples in Northern Europe. People feared that poisons in the leaves might be present in the fruit as well.

2 tomatoes = 1 Zone Block

Tomato-Zucchini Nibbles

Serves 4

Block size

1 Carbohydrate	1¼ cups zucchini, chopped fine
3 Carbohydrate	6 cups cherry tomatoes
4 Protein	1 cup cottage cheese
4 Fat	4 teaspoons slivered almonds, chopped
	¼ teaspoon garlic salt
	1 teaspoon snipped chives

In a saucepan, place zucchini and enough water to cover. Cook until tender. Remove from stove and cool. Using a knife, cut the tomatoes in half, then carefully cut out the inside of the tomato (or use a small melon baller to scoop it out) to create a tomato shell. If necessary, cut a little off the bottom of the tomatoes so that they will sit on a plate without moving. Using a blender, combine cooked zucchini, tomato pulp, cottage cheese, almonds, garlic salt, and chives. Blend until mixture is smooth. Fill tomatoes with cheese mixture by piping it out with a pastry bag. Arrange on serving plates and chill.

Wine   ☺ ☺

Yes, wine is a carbohydrate. You need to balance every glass with some protein and fat. Still, it's fine to include wine on the Zone Diet because several studies have established a link between wine consumption and lower rates of coronary artery disease. A landmark French study found that people who drank two 4-ounce glasses of wine daily had higher levels of high-density lipoprotein (HDL), the "good" cholesterol, than those who didn't. Another major study, in the United States, found that women who drank just one glass of wine a day had higher HDL levels than those who abstained. More good news: Japanese researchers discovered a compound in grape skin called resveratrol that lowers the amount of fat in the livers of rats, thus lowering overall cholesterol. They suspect it does the same in humans.

Although scientists once thought that only red wine conferred cardiovascular benefits, they now believe that white wine may be just as effective—based on recent research. Wine has another added benefit. Compounds in wine may promote absorption of calcium, phosphorus, magnesium, and zinc.

Did you know? Since ancient times, wine has been valued as a healing agent. The Jewish Talmud says, "Wine is the foremost of all medicines." Wine was one of the earliest anesthetics and was also used to disinfect wounds.

4 ounces of wine = 1 Zone Block

Wine and Cheese

Serves 1

Block size

1 Carbohydrate	4 ounces wine (or 6 ounces beer or 1 ounce distilled spirits)
1 Protein, 1 Fat	1 ounce cheese

Apples ☺

Everyone knows the saying "An apple a day keeps the doctor away," and apples do indeed provide a myriad of health benefits. Without a doubt apples are amazing for controlling blood sugar, which is a key point of the Zone Diet. Apples are a good source of soluble fiber, especially pectin, which helps control insulin levels by slowing the release of sugar into your bloodstream. Pectin also helps reduce cholesterol levels by lowering insulin secretion. Another type of soluble fiber in apples absorbs large amounts of water from the intestinal tract, which helps prevent constipation.

Although apples don't have an extremely high antioxidant capacity, whole fresh apples do contain caffeic or chlorogenic acid, which blocks cancer formation in lab animals given potent carcinogens.

Since apple trees are especially susceptible to worms, scale, and other insects, they are usually sprayed with pesticides several times during the growing season. Thus you should always wash apples carefully before eating them; some experts suggest even peeling them, especially if they have been waxed.

Did you know? Apples have been called "nature's toothbrush." Although they don't actually clean your teeth, they do promote dental hygiene. Biting and chewing stimulates your gums, and the sweetness of the apple causes an increased secretion of saliva, which reduces tooth decay by lowering the levels of bacteria in your mouth.

½ apple = 1 Zone Block

Cheddar-Apple "Galette"

Serves 1

Block size

	¼ to ⅛ cup purified water
	¼ teaspoon ground cinnamon
1 Carbohydrate	1 tablespoon raisins
3 Carbohydrate	1½ apples, such as Granny Smith or Fuji, halved, cored, and cut into eighths
4 Fat	4 walnut halves, chopped
4 Protein	4 ounces sharp low-fat cheddar cheese, grated

Preheat oven to 400°F. In a medium-size sauté pan that has a lid and can go into the oven, add water, cinnamon, raisins, and apples. Bring to a boil over high heat, then reduce to medium, cover, and simmer until apples are tender, about 6 to 10 minutes. Uncover pan and turn off heat. With a wooden spoon or spatula, form apple slices into a loose circle. Sprinkle with chopped walnuts and grated cheese. Transfer pan to oven and cook until cheese melts, about 3 to 5 minutes. Serve hot.

37

Celery   ☺

Celery may seem like just a stalk full of water, but it's actually a nutrition powerhouse—especially when it comes to fighting high blood pressure. One 8-inch stalk contains just a handful of calories and 120 mg of potassium, 5 percent of your minimum needs. Adding to this is an array of phytochemicals, one of which helps ward off high blood pressure. In a laboratory study, researchers saw a 10 percent drop in blood pressure in animals treated with the phytochemical, 3-n-butyl phthalide. Scientists theorize that this phytochemical helps control stress hormones in the body that trigger high blood pressure in some people.

Celery may also help reduce the risk of certain cancers. One compound in celery, called polyacetylene, destroys benzopyrene, a powerful carcinogen. This same compound is thought to reduce the production of "bad" eicosanoids, hormones that play a significant role in producing inflammation.

Did you know? Usually discarded, celery leaves are actually the most nutritious part of the plant, containing more calcium, iron, potassium, and vitamins A and C than the stalks. You can salvage the leaves to use in soups, salads, and other dishes enhanced by the flavor of celery.

2 cups of sliced celery = 1 Zone Block

Waldorf Salad

Serves 1

Block size

½ Carbohydrate	1 cup celery, sliced
½ Carbohydrate	½ apple, diced
1 Fat	1 teaspoon light mayonnaise
	1 pecan, crushed
1 Protein	1 ounce low-fat cheese

Combine and mix well.

Chickpeas   ☺

Often called garbanzo beans, chickpeas are a mainstay of Middle Eastern cuisine. Hummus (mashed chickpeas) and falafel balls (breaded and fried chickpeas—a real no-no on the Zone Diet) are served as commonly as salads. Tahini, an oily dressing also made from chickpeas, is the ketchup of Middle Eastern foods. With all these uses, I'd say that chickpeas are among the most versatile of legumes. They are extremely hard, however, and usually need to be soaked for at least a day or two in water before they can be used. Another option is to get canned chickpeas.

In terms of health benefits, chickpeas fall on the lower end of my carbohydrate list because they contain a hefty 27 carbohydrate grams to 7 grams of protein for a ⅔-cup serving—compared, for example, with black beans' 18 grams of carbohydrate to 7 grams of protein. Still, chickpeas confer many health benefits. Like other beans, chickpeas can keep insulin levels low due to their high fiber content. Research at Oxford University in England has shown that eating a diet rich in chickpeas and other legumes improved all aspects of diabetes control by lowering blood sugar and improving triglyceride levels. Other studies have found that ½ cup a day of beans can lower cholesterol levels by 19 percent.

Did you know? In the Jewish religion, chickpeas are customarily eaten to celebrate the birth of a new baby. Their small round shapes represent the continuing life cycle and fertility. You'll often find a bowl of chickpeas sitting next to the candies and cakes.

¼ cup of cooked chickpeas = 1 Zone Block

Hummus Deviled Eggs

Serves 1

Block size

1 Protein	2 hard-boiled eggs
1 Carbohydrate	¼ cup hummus
1 Fat	1 tablespoon slivered almonds

Cut the hard-boiled eggs in half, and discard the egg yolks. Fill each half of the hard-boiled egg white with the hummus. Sprinkle almonds on top.

Cucumbers ☺

With just a handful of calories per cup, cucumbers have always been a dieter's dream. What you may not know is that this crisp, refreshing vegetable also contains compounds called sterols, which have been shown to lower cholesterol in animals. The heaviest concentration of sterols is in the skin of the cucumber, so you shouldn't remove the peel before eating. (You can remove some of the waxy residue by scrubbing the cucumber with a brush while rinsing it with water.)

Cucumbers are also a great digestive aid and have a cleansing effect on the bowel. And they can improve the appearance of your skin.

Did you know? The old saying "cool as a cucumber" is literally true. Cucumbers actually have a cooling effect on the blood, which is why they're so refreshing on a hot summer day.

1½ cucumbers = 1 Zone Block

Cilantro Egg Salad

Serves 1

Block size

4 Protein	1 cup egg substitute
4 Fat	4 teaspoons reduced-fat mayonnaise
	⅛ teaspoon dry mustard
	½ teaspoon garlic, minced
	⅛ teaspoon cilantro
	Salt and pepper to taste
¼ Carbohydrate	¼ cup celery, minced
½ Carbohydrate	1 cup canned mushrooms, diced
¼ Carbohydrate	¼ cup onion, chopped
1 Carbohydrate	¼ cup kidney beans
½ Carbohydrate	5 cups lettuce
½ Carbohydrate	2 cups cucumber, sliced
1 Carbohydrate	2 cups tomatoes, diced

Pour egg substitute into a 10-ounce microwave-safe dish and cook on high (100 percent) setting for 1 to 2½ minutes or until set. Push cooked egg portions to center of the dish and continue cooking in 30-second intervals on high setting. When done, cool and dice cooked egg substitute. In a small bowl, blend mayonnaise and seasonings. Combine cooked egg substitute with the remaining ingredients in a medium-size bowl, toss to coat with mayonnaise, and serve.

40

Cherries   ☺

It's true that cherries contain fewer vitamins and minerals than larger members of their family such as plums, apricots, peaches, and nectarines. This is why cherries rank considerably lower on my Top 100 list. Still, they pack a powerfully sweet flavor in relatively few calories. A cup of cherries contains 140 calories and has 20 percent of the RDA for vitamin C as well as 500 mg of potassium. Cherries are also a good source of pectin, a soluble fiber that helps control blood cholesterol levels.

There's another reason cherries make my Top 100 list: Researchers recently discovered that cherries contain a powerful compound called ellagic acid. Ellagic acid interferes with natural and synthetic carcinogens, preventing these cancer-causing chemicals from turning healthy cells into malignancies. Folk healers used to recommend sour cherries to treat the arthritic symptoms caused by gout, and some alternative practitioners still prescribe cherries for that purpose, although this benefit remains unproven.

Did you know? From a nutritional standpoint, maraschino cherries are a far cry from cherries. They are made by bleaching the fruit in a sulfur dioxide brine, then toughening it with lime or calcium salt. The cherries are then dyed bright red, bathed in a sugary syrup, flavored, and packed in jars or canned. They're barely recognizable, either physically or nutritionally, as cherries.

8 cherries = 1 Zone Block

Melon-Cherry Protein Pops

Serves 4

Block size

	⅓ cup purified water, plus slightly more as needed to blend
4 Fat	4 teaspoons unsweetened almond or hazelnut butter, or 1⅓ teaspoons almond or hazelnut oil
	¼ teaspoon stevia extract powder
2 Carbohydrate	1⅓ cups honeydew melon, in chunks
4 Protein	1⅓ ounces unflavored protein powder (portion containing 28 grams protein)
	2 teaspoons pure vanilla or maple extract (nonalcohol, glycerine base)
2 Carbohydrate	¾ cup frozen, unsweetened, pitted cherries

Combine water, nut butter or oil, stevia powder, and melon in the blender and blend until smooth. Add protein powder and flavoring extract and blend until smooth. Scrape down the sides with a spatula as needed to mix in powder and dissolve lumps. Add cherries and blend, adding a little more water as needed to create a smooth

41

texture. Pour into eight Popsicle molds.* Affix the plastic tops with the built-in stick and holder. Freeze at least 3 to 4 hours, until firm. To serve, run warm water over the outside of each mold to loosen pops and allow for easy removal.

If you don't have plastic Popsicle molds, simply use small paper cups. Arrange the cups in a small cake pan, fill, and freeze 1 to 2 hours. When the mixture starts to ice up, insert a Popsicle stick into the center of each cup. Freeze until firm. Or forget the Popsicle idea altogether! Pour the mixture into four 8-ounce paper cups, freeze, and eat with a spoon.

Variations

Blueberry-Honeydew Protein Pops: Replace ¾ cup cherries with 1 cup fresh blueberries.

Cherry-Cantaloupe Pops: Replace 1⅓ cups honeydew melon with 1½ cups cantaloupe.

Yellow Squash ☺

Also called summer squash, yellow squash has a soft shell and tender flesh. The reason I don't include winter squashes (acorn, pumpkin, and butternut squash) in my Top 100 Zone Foods list is that they contain a high amount of carbohydrates (in the form of starch) and have a high glycemic index that can send your blood sugar levels soaring. Summer squash, on the other hand, is mostly water, but it also contains some important nutrients. A 1-cup serving provides 10 percent of the RDA for vitamin C, 15 mcg of folate, and small amounts of beta-carotene.

Yellow squash can be eaten raw. If it is cooked, stir-frying or steaming minimizes the loss of nutrients. The mild flavor goes nicely with stews, soups, and mixed vegetables, but squash can make some dishes watery. To avoid this problem, lightly salt the squash and place it on absorbent paper towels; rinse it before adding it to the recipe.

Did you know? Obviously you can eat a full-grown yellow squash, but you can also dine on the flowers, immature squash, and seeds—all of which are edible.

2 cups of cooked yellow squash = 1 Zone Block

Mexican-Style Yellow Squash with Beans and Soy Cheese

Serves 1

Block size

¼ Carbohydrate	⅛ cup + 1 tablespoon onion, chopped finely
	¼ teaspoon finely ground sea salt
	1 clove garlic, minced or pressed
½ Carbohydrate	1 cup zucchini, cut in half lengthwise, then in ½-inch rounds
½ Carbohydrate	1 cup yellow summer squash, cut in half lengthwise, then in ½-inch rounds
¼ Carbohydrate	½ red bell pepper, seeded, quartered, cut in thin strips
	½ to 1 teaspoon chili powder (according to taste)
	¼ teaspoon ground cumin
	¼ teaspoon dried basil, crumbled
	¼ teaspoon dried oregano, crumbled
	1 teaspoon tamari soy sauce
2 Carbohydrate	½ cup cooked, drained black or red beans
4 Protein	4 ounces nonfat mozzarella, Monterey Jack, or Colby-style soy cheese, grated

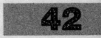

42

Salad:

¼ Carbohydrate	2½ cups shredded spring salad mix or red or green leaf lettuce
¼ Carbohydrate	½ cup cherry tomatoes, cut into halves

Dressing:

	2 to 3 teaspoons apple cider vinegar or lime juice
	1 teaspoon tamari or ume/umeboshi vinegar (Japanese plum vinegar)
	⅛ teaspoon ground red pepper
2 Fat	¼ teaspoon dry mustard (powder)
1 Fat	⅔ teaspoon extra-virgin or virgin olive oil
1 Fat	1 tablespoon light sour cream or mayonnaise
	3 olives, chopped

Spray a nonstick 9- to 10-inch skillet with cooking spray, add onion, and sauté. When onion begins to soften, add sea salt to draw out moisture. Add garlic, zucchini, summer squash, and bell pepper, stirring for 1 to 2 minutes after each addition. Add spices and tamari. (If using an electric range, you may need to add about 2 tablespoons of water to prevent sticking and burning.) Cover skillet and bring to steam over medium-high heat. Reduce heat and simmer for 15 to 18 minutes, until vegetables are almost tender and juicy. Top with beans but do not stir. Cover and simmer for 4 to 5 minutes. Sprinkle cheese on top. Remove pan from heat source. Arrange salad greens or lettuce and tomatoes on a large dinner plate. Mix dressing ingredients, then pour over salad. Transfer squash and beans dish to dinner plate and serve.

Grapes   ☺

You've no doubt heard about the health benefits of drinking red wine, so it should be no great surprise that grapes confer the same benefits, since they are the main component of wine. In terms of vitamins, grapes are not much to speak of; they have only modest amounts of fiber, potassium, and vitamin C, and at 100 calories a cup are more caloric than many other fruits. Grapes, though, have a host of hidden phytochemicals called flavonoids, which can help fight heart disease by lowering cholesterol levels. One flavonoid in particular, called resveratrol, has been shown to help protect against arterial wall damage by "bad" (LDL) cholesterol. Contained in the grape's skin, resveratrol is found in grapes, grape juice, grape jelly, and wine.

Grapes may also be potent against viruses and tumors because of their high concentration of another compound called tannin. Canadian researchers found that grapes could effectively kill off disease-causing viruses in test tubes. When they added grape extract to vials containing polio and herpes simplex viruses, the viruses were completely inactivated. Whether grapes destroy viruses inside the body isn't known, but tannin can get into the bloodstream and possibly protect against viruses. What's more, grapes also contain caffeic acid, a powerful chemical that has been shown to prevent cancer in animals.

Did you know? In 1928 Johanna Brandt, an author from South Africa, wrote a book, *The Grape Cure,* in which she claims that grapes cured her abdominal cancer. The "grape cure" was instantly popular on several continents and still is in parts of Europe.

½ cup of grapes = 1 Zone Block

Cheese and Grape Snack

Serves 1

Block size

1 Protein	1 ounce part-skim mozzarella string cheese
1 Carbohydrate	½ cup grapes
1 Fat	6 peanuts

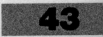

43

Kidney Beans ☺

One of the most popular and versatile legumes is the kidney bean, whether you're mixing some into chili or sprinkling some on your salad. Like other legumes, kidney beans are rich in B vitamins, zinc, potassium, magnesium, calcium, and iron. They are also rich in soluble fiber, which can help stabilize blood sugar levels by slowing the entry of glucose into your bloodstream.

Beans have been dubbed "gourmet preventive medicine," and medical research continues to document their health benefits. Early research at Oxford University showed that a diet high in legumes improved all aspects of diabetes, including lowered blood sugars and improved triglyceride levels. An added bonus: improving triglyceride levels helps prevent the heart attacks and strokes that occur three to four times more often in diabetic than in nondiabetic individuals.

Did you know? Kidney beans are named for their color and shape. They are a favorite dish in the Turkish cuisine passed down from the Ottoman cuisine. Appetizers and side dishes containing kidney beans are called *meze*.

¼ cup of cooked kidney beans = 1 Zone Block

Red-Bean Chili

Serves 1

Block size

4 Fat	1⅓ teaspoons olive oil
¼ Carbohydrate	½ medium onion, chopped
¼ Carbohydrate	½ medium green bell pepper, seeded and chopped
	1 teaspoon chili powder
	½ teaspoon ground cumin
	¼ teaspoon sea or regular salt
	¼ teaspoon garlic powder, or 1 clove garlic, chopped
2 Protein	⅔ cup soybean hamburger crumbles (found in the freezer section, usually with the breakfast meats)
	½ cup purified water
1½ Carbohydrate	1¼ cups canned crushed tomatoes
2 Carbohydrate	½ cup canned kidney beans, drained and rinsed
2 Protein	2 ounces low-fat Monterey Jack or soy cheese, grated or thinly sliced

In a large nonstick sauté pan with a cover, heat oil over medium heat. Sauté onion and green pepper in oil for 5 minutes or until onion turns translucent. Add chili powder, cumin, salt, and garlic. Cook another 2 minutes.

44

Add soybean hamburger crumbles and water. Stir in tomatoes and kidney beans. Cover and simmer 10 to 30 minutes to blend flavors. Serve in a bowl, sprinkled with grated cheese.

Leeks   ☺

Leeks are closely related to onions, as their appearance and taste suggest. You can eat the entire leek, but most people choose to eat only the white fleshy base and tender inner leaves. Leeks are a great source of vitamin C, an immune boosting anti-oxidant that also helps prevent the buildup of plaque on the walls of your arteries. Leeks also contain small amounts of niacin and calcium and are naturally low in calories. You can use leeks in a wide range of dishes, from leek quiche made with steamed leeks, egg whites, and plain yogurt to grilled leeks and mixed vegetables brushed lightly with olive oil.

Caveat: Leeks are a natural sandtrap. Their layered structure collects large amounts of gritty sand and garden soil. They need to be washed carefully, layer by layer, before they are cooked.

Did you know? Leeks are the national symbol of Wales. Men parade in the streets with leek-bedecked hats on a special holiday.

1 cup of cooked leeks = 1 Zone Block

Grilled Sole with Leeks

Serves 1

Block size

4 Fat	1⅓ teaspoons olive oil
3 Carbohydrate	3 cups sliced leeks
4 Protein	6 ounces fillet of sole
1 Carbohydrate	4 ounces white wine (optional)
	1 teaspoon minced garlic
	1 shallot, minced
	1 teaspoon dill
	Salt to taste
	Pepper to taste
	½ teaspoon lemon herb
	seasoning

Preheat oven to 375°F. Brush a medium-size baking dish with the olive oil. Layer bottom of dish with leeks. Place sole on top. In a medium bowl, combine wine, garlic, shallot, dill, salt, and pepper. Gently pour wine mixture into baking dish. Sprinkle with lemon herb seasoning. Tightly cover baking dish and place in oven. Bake for 25 to 30 minutes and serve.

45

Mushrooms   ☺

You can't call it a vegetable or a fruit. A mushroom is actually a fungus, one of the most primitive life forms around. Mushrooms are a staple in many Asian diets, and Japanese scientists have taken the lead in studying their health benefits. They have found that mushrooms may boost immune system functioning, helping you fight cancer, infections, and autoimmune diseases such as lupus and rheumatoid arthritis. The reason may be mushrooms' high content of glutamic acid, an amino acid that plays a role in fighting infections and strengthening the immune system.

Mushrooms may also help lower high blood pressure as well as blood cholesterol levels. Researchers from the University of Dhaka in Bangladesh gave animals that were genetically engineered to develop hypertension, especially when given salt, dried mushrooms mixed in with their regular food for about two months. The animals' blood pressure and cholesterol levels dropped significantly compared with those of animals that ate a mushroom-free diet. Rich in potassium and low in calories, mushrooms enhance the flavor of a variety of dishes. Try dried mushrooms in soups, stews, and casseroles. Add your favorite variety to omelettes, stews, and casseroles.

Did you know? In Oriental folklore, mushrooms are highly regarded as a longevity tonic. In fact, they are the symbol for the Chinese god of longevity. The Chinese black fungus is used to treat headaches and prevent heart attacks. In Japan, the basidiomycete fungus has been used as a folk remedy for cancer.

2 cups of cooked mushrooms = 1 Zone Block

Mediterranean Mushroom Gratin

Serves 1

Block size	
	3 to 4 tablespoons purified water
	1 clove garlic, minced
	½ teaspoon dried oregano
	⅛ teaspoon ground black pepper
½ Carbohydrate	1 small yellow onion, chopped
¼ Carbohydrate	½ medium red bell pepper, seeded, diced
¼ Carbohydrate	½ medium yellow bell pepper, seeded, diced
⅓ Carbohydrate	1⅓ cups cremini or button mushrooms, thinly sliced
⅓ Carbohydrate	1⅓ cups broccoli florets and stems, peeled and finely chopped
⅓ Carbohydrate	1⅓ cups cauliflower florets
1 Carbohydrate	1 medium carrot, peeled, thinly sliced
4 Fat	12 olives, pitted, sliced
	Scant bread crumbs
4 Protein	4 ounces soy cheese, grated
1 Carbohydrate	½ cup grapes

Preheat oven to 400°F. In a sauté pan that has a cover and can go into the oven, put water, garlic, oregano, and pepper. Stir in onion, red and yellow peppers, mushrooms,

broccoli, cauliflower florets, and carrot. Bring to a boil over high heat, then reduce to low heat and simmer, covered, for about 6 to 10 minutes, or until vegetables are tender. (Add water if needed.) Remove lid from skillet and add olives. Sprinkle scant bread crumbs and grated cheese onto vegetables. Place skillet, uncovered, in oven and bake until cheese melts, about 4 to 6 minutes. Use spatula to transfer vegetable melt to serving plate. Garnish with grapes.

Navy Beans   ☺

Also called haricots, Great Northern, or cannellini, navy beans are probably the most widely used of all common beans. They are so named because they were once a fixture in the navy mess hall. Beans are a great way to reduce your insulin levels if they are used as part of a balanced Zone Diet. Researchers at the University of Kentucky found that diabetics can lower their fasting blood sugar levels and reduce their cholesterol by adding 8 ounces of beans to their daily diet. Your body digests beans more slowly because of their high soluble fiber content, which helps you avoid a sudden surge in blood glucose. This soluble fiber also helps reduce blood cholesterol levels.

Navy beans, however, are very dense in carbohydrates—27 grams in ⅔ cup. For this reason, you can't eat them in limitless amounts. Stick to a single serving size and remember to balance them with protein and a small amount of fat.

Did you know? The history of navy beans dates back to the Sunday dinners of the pilgrims. They are used today to make Boston baked beans.

¼ cup of cooked navy beans = 1 Zone Block

Beef and Navy Bean Stew

Serves 2

Block size

4 Carbohydrate	1 cup cooked navy beans*
1 Carbohydrate	1½ cups onion, diced
8 Fat	2⅔ teaspoons olive oil, divided
1 Carbohydrate	½ cup tomato puree
	⅛ teaspoon Worcestershire sauce
	½ cup beef stock
	½ teaspoon chili powder
	⅛ teaspoon dried basil
	⅛ teaspoon curry powder
	⅛ teaspoon dried oregano
	Salt and pepper to taste
2 Carbohydrate	1 cup salsa
8 Protein	8 ounces beef (eye of round), sliced ⅛ inch thick, then diced

In a saucepan, cook beans and onion in 2 teaspoons oil until tender, then add tomato puree, Worcestershire sauce, beef stock, spices, and salsa. Continue cooking vegetable mixture over medium heat until hot. While the vegetables are cooking add remaining oil to nonstick sauté pan and stir-fry beef until cooked. Add beef to vegetables and simmer for 5 minutes. Place an equal amount in two soup bowls and serve.

Always rinse canned beans before using.

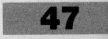

47

Onions   ☺

Recognizing the potential health benefits of the onion, the National Cancer Institute has placed it pretty high up on its list of foods being investigated for cancer-fighting properties, even though its anti-oxidative capacity is relatively low. The onion first attracted the attention of the scientific community in 1989 when a study was published in the *Journal of the National Cancer Institute* finding that people who ate the largest amount of onions had the lowest rates of stomach cancer. Other research has shown that a variety of chemicals in onion can halt the growth of malignant cells in test tubes.

Onions contain flavonoids, including quercetin, that appear to inhibit the growth of estrogen-sensitive cells, which often give rise to breast cancers. Onions may also have a beneficial effect on cholesterol levels, according to some studies. Researchers found that people who eat an onion a day can raise their "good" (HDL) cholesterol. An added benefit of onions: a recently discovered sulfur compound in onions may prevent the biochemical chain of events that leads to asthma and inflammatory reactions. Onions also contain compounds that may work to alleviate diabetes. Indian researchers found that boiled onions caused drops in blood sugar in diabetics who had been given glucose. What's more, Egyptian pharmacists isolated a compound in onions, diphenylamine, and found it more potent than the diabetes drug tolbutamide in lowering blood sugar in laboratory rabbits.

Did you know? Onions have been used for centuries as a health remedy to treat everything from dysentery and bloating to high blood pressure and lack of sexual desire. A 1927 medical journal calls onions "blood purifiers, sedatives, expectorants . . . beneficial in cases of insomnia, general nervous irritability, coughs and bronchial troubles."

½ cup of cooked or 1½ cups of chopped raw onions = 1 Zone Block

Barbecue Beef with Onions

Serves 2

Block size

8 Fat	2⅔ teaspoons olive oil, divided
8 Protein	8 ounces beef (eye of round) in ⅛-inch slices
4 Carbohydrate	2 cups tomato puree
	1 teaspoon Worcestershire sauce
	1 teaspoon cider vinegar
	½ teaspoon chili powder
	⅛ teaspoon dried oregano
	¼ teaspoon minced garlic
4 Carbohydrate	4 cups onion, in half rings
	2 tablespoons beef stock
	2 tablespoons white wine vinegar

In nonstick sauté pan with a cover, add ⅔ teaspoon oil and sauté the beef until browned. Then add tomato puree, Worcestershire sauce, cider vinegar, chili powder, oregano, and garlic, cover, and simmer for 5 minutes until a sauce forms. While the beef is simmering, in another nonstick sauté pan add remaining oil and onion. Cook onion until tender. Add the onion, beef stock, and white wine vinegar to the beef mixture. Cover sauté pan and cook 10 minutes, stirring occasionally to blend flavors. Place an equal amount on two lunch plates or in soup bowls and serve.

48

Peaches ☺

Although not quite as packed with nutrition as its cousin the nectarine, a peach still packs a strong nutritional punch. A medium-size peach contains an impressive 2 grams of dietary fiber, 470 IU of beta-carotene (almost 10 percent of the RDA), a touch of potassium, and let's not forget, a succulent sweet taste. All for a mere 35 calories, which doesn't add up to many insulin-triggering carbohydrates.

You can find peaches from late May through mid-October. Choose ones that feel heavy, indicating that they are juicy, and that have a sweet odor. Avoid those that are pale yellow or greenish, which means they are underripe, not as sweet, and have fewer disease-fighting phytochemicals.

Did you know? The Chinese philosopher Confucius refers to peaches in his writings, which date back to the fifth century B.C. The "Persian apple," as the peach was called, was introduced to Greece and Rome from China in around A.D. 100. It was then introduced to northern Europe, where it soon became the most popular fruit.

1 peach = 1 Zone Block

Sweet and Spicy Peaches

Serves 2

Block size

5 Carbohydrate	5 peaches, peeled, pitted, and sliced
	1 tablespoon vanilla extract (nonalcohol, glycerine base)
	⅛ teaspoon allspice
1 Carbohydrate	2 teaspoons brown sugar
2 Protein	2 envelopes Knox Unflavored Gelatin
	½ cup purified water
4 Protein	2 ounces protein powder (28 grams of protein)
2 Protein, 2 Carbohydrate	1 cup plain low-fat yogurt, lightly heated
8 Fat	8 teaspoons almonds, sliced

In a saucepan, gently heat peaches, vanilla extract, allspice, brown sugar, gelatin, and water until hot. In a mixing bowl, combine protein powder with yogurt. Place yogurt and protein powder mixture into two serving bowls, top with heated fruit and sliced almonds, and serve.

49

Pears   ☺

Called the "butter fruit" by many Europeans, referring to its smooth texture, a pear makes a great snack, especially if preventing constipation is on your mind. A pear contains a whopping 3 grams of fiber. Some of the fiber is the soluble pectin, which helps control blood cholesterol levels. The bulk of the fiber, though, is insoluble, which promotes regularity and may offer some protection against colon cancer. One pear also contains 10 percent of the RDA for vitamin C and a moderate amount of potassium.

Most of the vitamin C is concentrated in the skin of the fruit, so you should eat pears unpeeled. What's more, canned pears lose most of their vitamin C due to the combined effect of peeling and heating. They are also usually high in sugar if they are packed in a heavy syrup, so I strongly recommend that you stick to fresh pears.

Did you know? In the eighteenth and nineteenth centuries, advances in pear cultivation greatly improved their taste and quality. In 1850 pears were so popular in France that the fruit was celebrated in song and verse, and the wealthy held friendly contests to see who could grow the best specimen.

½ **pear = 1 Zone Block**

Poached Pears with Cheese

Serves 8

Block size

1 Carbohydrate	4 ounces Johannesburg Riesling Wine
	½ teaspoon orange extract (nonalcohol, glycerine base)
	½ teaspoon lemon extract (nonalcohol, glycerine base)
½ Carbohydrate	2 teaspoons cornstarch
6 Carbohydrate	3 pears, halved, cored, and sliced in thin strips
	Dash of ground cloves
8 Protein	2 cups low-fat cottage cheese
8 Fat	8 teaspoons almonds, slivered
½ Carbohydrate	¼ cup blueberries

In a small nonstick sauté pan, combine wine, extracts, and cornstarch. (Mix cornstarch in wine before adding to sauté pan.) Add pears to the sauté pan and bring to a simmer. Simmer for 3 to 5 minutes, stirring frequently, until the pears soften and the juices reduce and thicken. As the mixture cooks, add cloves. Divide cottage cheese into the bottom of eight serving bowls. Place warm pears on top of cottage cheese. Sprinkle with almonds and blueberries and serve.

50

Tangerines ☺

I'll be the first to admit that the tangerine doesn't quite stack up against the orange. Ounce for ounce, an orange has twice the amount of vitamin C. Still, a medium-size tangerine meets 50 percent of your RDA for this anti-oxidant. What's more, tangerines are richer in beta-carotene (a precursor of vitamin A) than any other citrus fruit. They also provide plenty of potassium and pectin, a soluble fiber that helps lower blood cholesterol and plays a role in helping to maintain insulin levels.

Tangerines also contain a number of disease-fighting phytochemicals, including flavonoids, which help protect against cancer, and terpenes, which reduce the amount of cholesterol produced by your body.

Did you know? A tangerine is actually a type of mandarin orange. It is from China, but as it moved into other tropical and subtropical areas, it was crossed with other citrus fruits to produce a variety of hybrids, including tangelos (a cross between a tangerine and a grapefruit) and tangors (a cross between a tangerine and an orange).

1 tangerine = 1 Zone Block

Tangerine-Strawberry Dream Smoothie

Serves 4

Block size

1 Protein, 1 Carbohydrate	1 cup 1% milk
1 Protein, 1 Carbohydrate	½ cup plain low-fat yogurt
1 Carbohydrate	1 cup strawberries
1 Carbohydrate	½ cup tangerine segments
4 Fat	4 teaspoons almonds, slivered
2 Protein	14 grams protein powder

Place all ingredients except protein powder in blender. Blend until smooth, then add protein powder. Pour into four glasses and serve immediately.

Zucchini ☺

Packed with potassium and only 15 calories per ½ cup cooked, zucchini will never lead you astray nutritionally. Potassium and the fiber found in zucchini can play a role in controlling blood pressure. In fact, a famous clinical trial, called Dietary Approaches to Stop Hypertension (DASH), found that participants with high blood pressure who ate 8 to 10 servings of vegetables and fruits every day—a third less than you get on the Zone Diet—experienced a drop in blood pressure similar to that seen with medications.

Small zucchini are great for stir-fries and soups and grated in muffins and breads or in stews and casseroles. You can also grill zucchini; just place them in boiling water for a few minutes to blanch them, and marinate them before grilling. For larger zucchini, stuff them with barley and mushrooms for a gourmet appetizer or side dish.

Did you know? The Texan wild marrow, *Cucurbita texana,* with small hard-skinned fruits, is viewed as an ancestor of the zucchini. This small-seeded ancient vegetable was cultivated in Mexico around 7000 to 5000 B.C. As soon as 50 years after the discovery of the Americas, numerous cultivated varieties, including the zucchini, were distributed in Europe.

2 cups of cooked zucchini = 1 Zone Block

Ratatouille with "Sausage"

Serves 1

Block size

Block	Ingredient
4 Fat	1½ teaspoons olive oil
¼ Carbohydrate	⅓ cup onion, chopped
	½ teaspoon finely ground sea salt
	1 clove garlic, minced or pressed
¼ Carbohydrate	½ cup eggplant, peeled and diced
½ Carbohydrate	1 cup zucchini, cut in half lengthwise, then cut into ½-inch-wide slices
¼ Carbohydrate	½ yellow or red bell pepper, seeded and diced
1 Carbohydrate	½ cup tomato sauce bottled or canned, unsweetened, oil-free, or 1½ cups fresh tomato, chopped
	¼ teaspoon ground black pepper
	¼ teaspoon each dried basil, oregano, and thyme, crumbled between your fingers
1½ Protein, 1 Carbohydrate	2 Light Life Lean Links, cubed
¼ Carbohydrate	1 cup cauliflower, cut into bite-size florets
	Purified water to steam
¾ Carbohydrate	½ cup asparagus, sliced into 1-inch lengths

52

Topping:

2½ Protein   2½ ounces low-fat mozzarella, cheddar, or Colby-style soy cheese, grated

Add oil to a 1-quart saucepan or deep skillet and heat over medium setting. Add onion, then sea salt. Stir and cook for about 3 minutes, until tender. Add garlic, eggplant, zucchini, and bell pepper, stirring after each addition. Cook for about 2 to 3 minutes. Add tomato sauce, pepper, basil, oregano, and thyme. Top with sliced "sausages" but do not stir. Cover, reduce heat to medium-low, and simmer for about 15 minutes, until vegetables are tender. Meanwhile, place cauliflower in a steamer in a 2-quart pot with 1 to 2 inches of purified water. Top with asparagus. Cover and bring to a boil over medium-high heat. Reduce heat to medium and steam for 5 to 7 minutes or until vegetables are fork-tender. Transfer cauliflower and asparagus to a large soup bowl or dinner plate with sides. Remove lid from ratatouille and continue cooking for another 5 minutes to reduce liquid. Sprinkle with grated soy cheese and remove from heat. Serve ratatouille over steamed vegetables.

Note: Make a double batch to serve two people or one person for two days in a row. (If making a larger batch, add the cheese to individual portions at the table.) Store the leftovers in a jar, then reheat the next day.

Variation

Omit sausages and increase soy cheese to 4 ounces.

PROTEIN

Haddock   ☺ ☺ ☺

Like other fish, haddock is an excellent source of B-complex vitamins and essential trace minerals, including potassium, iron, phosphorus, copper, iodine, manganese, cobalt, and selenium. Recent studies indicate that a meal or two of fish each week may also help reduce blood cholesterol levels. Like cod, its white-fish cousin, haddock contains a modest amount of heart-healthy Omega-3 fatty acids, though not nearly as much as salmon.

Haddock offers high-quality protein with fewer calories than a similar-size portion of meat. Consider this: haddock and ground beef are both about 18 percent protein, but the haddock has only about 22 calories per ounce, while regular ground beef has about 80 calories per ounce. When buying fresh haddock, look for bright glossy skin, clear bulging eyes, tight scales, and firm flesh. You shouldn't smell any fishy odor, just a clean briny ammonia smell.

Did you know? Just 30 years ago, haddock was so plentiful in the coastal waters off Cape Cod that fishermen would often give the fish away to local residents who asked. Now haddock is an endangered species in that area, and the U.S. government has placed tight controls on the amount of haddock that can be fished from the waters. Haddock, now shipped from Norway and Iceland, is a pricey import and no longer a bargain purchase for New England residents.

1½ ounces of haddock = 1 Zone Block

Poached Haddock with Hot Green Beans and Artichokes

Serves 4

Block size

	1 cup purified water
	½ cup onion, sliced thin
	2 cups 2% milk
	¼ teaspoon sea salt
	Pepper

12 Protein   4 haddock fillets, each weighing 5 ounces for a total of approximately 20 ounces

Parsley to garnish

Sauce:

3 Fat   1 teaspoon butter

1½ tablespoons flour

1 cup poaching liquid

Optional: 20 green grapes

Marinade:

3 tablespoons lemon juice

⅛ cup red wine vinegar

¼ cup olive oil

11 Carbohydrate   16 cups green beans
1 Carbohydrate   1 cup drained artichoke hearts
9 Fat   1 tablespoon olive oil

½ cup chopped parsley

¼ cup chopped chives

Optional: 2 tablespoons chopped pimiento

53

In a large skillet, preferably stainless steel or enameled cast iron, bring the water and onion to a boil. Add the milk, salt, and pepper, and add the fish fillets. Reduce the heat and cook for 5 or 6 minutes. Turn off the heat and remove the fillets to a warm platter.

Over medium heat, reduce the poaching liquid by half. Meanwhile, prepare the sauce. In a small saucepan, over medium heat, melt the butter. Add the flour and cook for a minute, while whisking, to cook the flour. Whisk in half the cup of poaching liquid. The sauce will thicken immediately. Add the rest of the liquid and whisk well. Add green grapes and return the sauce to a boil. Adjust the seasoning and serve the sauce with Hot Green Beans and Artichokes over the fish and garnish with parsley.

Mix marinade ingredients together. Toss green beans and artichoke hearts in marinade. Keep in a covered glass dish in the refrigerator until ready to cook.

Drain off as much of the marinade as possible. Heat the olive oil in a large skillet. Toss beans and artichoke hearts until heated through (about 3 or 4 minutes). Add parsley and chives. You can add chopped pimiento for color at the last minute.

Cod   ☺ ☺ ☺

Icelanders have one of the longest lifespans of any na-
tionality in the Western world. They may owe their
longevity to cod. While most Americans are eating
burgers and fries, Icelanders are gorging on cod, which
is incredibly low in saturated fat and calories. One
4-ounce serving has just 118 calories and a minute 37
mg of cholesterol. Cod are also environmentally correct:
they are relatively pollutant-free since they are both low
in fat (which stores contaminants like PCB) and caught
offshore away from polluted waters. Cod is also rich in
vitamin B_{12}, which is needed by the body to prevent pernicious anemia, nerve problems, and muscle weakness.

Cod is one of the best high-quality proteins. This is
because it contains very low levels of saturated fats and
larger amounts of the heart-healthy Omega-3 fatty
acids—but not nearly as much as salmon and other
dark-fleshed fish like mackerel or sardines. Cod,
though, is still an excellent source of a complete protein
that is naturally low in fat.

Did you know? For 1,000 years cod was a trading commodity central to Europe's development. Fishing for cod
on the Atlantic seas and continuing to head westward,
the Basques of northwestern Iberia and then the Norse
discovered America well before Columbus. Later cod
became a key player in the slave trade: the best dried
cod was traded in Europe for merchandise, which was
then traded for humans in Africa. Lower grades of cod,
still highly nutritious, were sold to feed West Indian
plantation slaves.

1½ ounces of cod = 1 Zone Block

Oven-Wrapped Codfish

Serves 1

Block size

3 Protein	4½-ounce codfish fillet
	Vegetable spray
	Onion to taste, chopped
	Freshly ground pepper to taste
	Squirt of lemon juice
	Sprinkling of Parmesan cheese
1 Carbohydrate	3 cups shredded lettuce
	½ cup green pepper
	½ cup cucumber
	1 tomato
2 Carbohydrate	1 apple

Preheat oven to 425°F. Tear off a good-size piece of foil. Spray the center lightly with vegetable spray. Put the fish in the center of the foil with the onion, pepper, lemon juice, and cheese. Fold foil over the fish, leaving space around the fish. Carefully turn up and seal the sides and the middle so that juices don't leak out. Bake for 18 minutes. When done, open the foil carefully to prevent steam burns. Mix lettuce, green peppers, cucumber, and tomato for a tossed salad. Serve apple for dessert.

54

Crabmeat   ☺ ☺ ☺

Shellfish has received somewhat of a bad rap in recent years, and you might be surprised to see crabmeat on my list of Top 100 Zone Foods. In fact, crab and other shellfish are good sources of chromium; this mineral improves insulin's ability to store blood sugar, which helps keep your insulin levels on a more even keel because you are not forcing the pancreas to pump out more. Chromium also helps to raise the levels of "good" (HDL) cholesterol, which can reduce your risk of heart disease and stroke. In addition, crab and shellfish contain plentiful amounts of selenium, a powerhouse mineral that works as an anti-oxidant to neutralize carcinogenic substances that can turn healthy cells into cancerous ones. Studies have shown that test patients with the highest blood selenium levels have the lowest cancer rates. Selenium also helps protect against heart and circulatory diseases.

Your best bet is to purchase live crabs whenever possible. Crabs should be alert and brandish their pinchers when poked. Soft-shell crabs should be translucent and completely soft. Crabs should have a fresh saltwater aroma; avoid those that smell sour or extremely fishy. Thawed, cooked crab should also be odor-free, and thawed only on the day of sale. You can also buy vacuum-packed crabmeat, either fresh or frozen.

Did you know? The crab is one of the oldest species on earth. The horseshoe crab dates back more than 200 million years and is literally a living fossil.

1½ ounces of crabmeat = 1 Zone Block

Florentine Crab Salad

Serves 1

Block size

4 Fat	1⅓ teaspoons olive oil
4 Protein	6 ounces canned crabmeat
¼ Carbohydrate	¼ cup scallions, sliced (white and green parts)
¼ Carbohydrate	1 cup mushrooms, sliced
1 Carbohydrate	¼ cup cooked kidney beans, rinsed
	1 tablespoon balsamic vinegar
	⅛ teaspoon Worcestershire sauce
	⅛ teaspoon celery salt
	½ teaspoon garlic, minced
	2 teaspoons white Zinfandel wine
	⅛ teaspoon chili powder
	Pepper to taste
1 Carbohydrate	½ cup Zoned Herb Dressing (see page 68)
½ Carbohydrate	5 cups raw spinach, stems removed
½ Carbohydrate	2 cups shredded cabbage (or coleslaw mix)
½ Carbohydrate	½ apple

Heat oil in a medium-size nonstick sauté pan. Add crab, scallions, mushrooms, kidney beans, vinegar, Worcestershire sauce, celery salt, garlic, wine, chili powder, and

55

pepper. Sauté until cooked through. Stir in Zoned Herb Dressing. Simmer 3 to 5 minutes. In a medium-size bowl, combine spinach and cabbage. Top with crab mixture and serve. Have apple for dessert.

Egg Whites (or Egg Substitutes) ☺ ☺ ☺

Egg whites contain all the great nutrition of eggs without any of the damaging cholesterol or saturated fat found in egg yolks. Egg whites also contain none of the Omega-6 fatty acid, known as arachidonic acid, that causes the production of the "bad" eicosanoids, the hormones that trigger chronic disease conditions like heart disease, cancer, and diabetes. Only the yolk contains this fatty acid. Egg whites are an excellent source of protein and vitamin B₁₂, which is essential for proper nerve function.

As long as you like your eggs scrambled or in omelette form, egg substitutes are a great option. Along with vitamin B₁₂, both egg whites and egg substitutes contain folate, riboflavin, and vitamin A. One advantage of egg substitutes over plain egg whites is that they are pasteurized (heat-treated), so there is no risk of food poisoning from the salmonella found in raw eggs. For any recipe that calls for uncooked eggs, you can safely use egg substitutes.

Did you know? Americans tend to think of chicken eggs as the only eggs that are eaten. In other countries, though, quail, duck, and goose eggs are more commonly found in refrigerators.

2 egg whites or ¼ cup of egg substitute = 1 Zone Block

Huevos Rancheros

Serves 1

Block size

4 Fat	1⅓ teaspoons olive oil
1 Protein	1 whole egg
1 Protein	2 egg whites
1 Carbohydrate	½ cup each of chopped onion, green pepper, and tomato to taste
	Chili powder to taste
1 Carbohydrate	1 corn tortilla
2 Protein	2 ounces low-fat cheese
	1 tablespoon chopped cilantro
1 Carbohydrate	1 cup strawberries served on the side
1 Carbohydrate	½ cup blueberries served on the side

Heat oil in a skillet. Scramble egg, egg whites, chopped vegetables, and chili powder. Place scrambled eggs in tortilla and top with cheese and cilantro. Roll up tortilla. Serve strawberries and blueberries on the side.

56

Lobster   ☺ ☺ ☺

You may have heard that shellfish like lobster isn't nutritionally sound because it raises your cholesterol levels. Forget about this myth. Lobster is actually a wise choice if you skip the dip in melted butter. (Dip it in some lemon juice and olive oil instead.) Lobster actually protects your arteries and blood vessels by significantly lowering "bad" (LDL) cholesterol. It also contains a moderate dose of Omega-3 fatty acids, which can help prevent dangerous blood clots in your arteries and may be protective against a long list of diseases such as rheumatoid arthritis, asthma, psoriasis, and cancer.

A 3½-ounce serving of boiled lobster provides 19 grams of protein and 1.5 grams of fat. Lobster is a great source of vitamin B_{12}, which is needed to make red blood cells and prevent pernicious anemia. It's also a good source of zinc, necessary to keep your immune system functioning. Lobster also contains some folate, magnesium, potassium, and calcium.

Did you know? Lobster can boost your mood and mental performance. According to research performed at MIT, lobster and other shellfish deliver large supplies of an amino acid called tyrosine to the brain. Tyrosine is used to produce two energizing brain chemicals called dopamine and norepinephrine.

1½ ounces of lobster = 1 Zone Block

Lobster Salad

Serves 1

Block size

3 Protein	4½ ounces lobster
3 Fat	1 tablespoon light mayonnaise
2 Carbohydrate	1 mini-pita pocket or 1 piece rye bread*
1 Carbohydrate	½ orange

Mix seafood and mayonnaise. Stuff in mini-pita pocket. Serve with the orange.

*Or eliminate the bread and place the seafood on top of a tossed salad. If you use the mayonnaise with the seafood, don't use salad dressing. Or substitute 1 tablespoon olive oil and vinegar dressing and hold the mayonnaise.

Mackerel   ☺ ☺ ☺

In terms of Zone quality, mackerel is one of the best protein choices you can find. It contains a heaping amount of long-chain Omega-3 fatty acids—2.1 grams per 4-ounce serving. This is an amazing amount, considering that research from the National Heart and Lung Institute found that just 1 gram of long-chain Omega-3 fatty acids may reduce the risk of heart disease in men by as much as 40 percent. (Although the research was done only in men, I would hazard a guess that women reap the same health benefits.)

In addition to its mega amount of long-chain Omega-3 fatty acids, mackerel also contains 10 percent of the RDA for calcium and is a good source of vitamin D, which aids the absorption of calcium. It's also rich in the anti-oxidant vitamins A and E. Adding to this trove of nutrients, mackerel is packed with B vitamins, and is an excellent source of niacin, thiamine, B_{12}, and riboflavin.

Did you know? According to the historian Seamus Fitzgerald, the city of Baltimore became a major landing place for the export of mackerel to England during the nineteenth century. In fact, he suggests that the now defunct Baltimore Railway Station and the nearby Baltimore Fishery School, now in ruins, disappeared with the vanished and largely forgotten mackerel industry.

1½ ounces of mackerel = 1 Zone Block

Smoked Mackerel with Radish and Endive

Serves 1

Block size

4 Protein	6 ounces smoked mackerel
½ Carbohydrate	2 cups radishes, sliced
½ Carbohydrate	1 cup red and green pepper strips
½ Carbohydrate	¾ cup red onion, diced
1 Carbohydrate	½ Granny Smith apple, diced
½ Carbohydrate	5 cups Belgian endive, chopped
4 Fat	1⅓ teaspoons olive oil
	2 teaspoons cider vinegar
	Horseradish, grated (bottled or fresh to taste)
1 Carbohydrate	½ cup Zoned Herb Dressing (see page 68)
	¼ teaspoon dill weed
	⅛ teaspoon dry mustard
	Salt and pepper to taste

Combine mackerel, radishes, peppers, onion, apple, and endive in a medium-size salad bowl. In a blender combine oil, vinegar, horseradish, Zoned Herb Dressing, herbs, and salt and pepper. Pulse until well mixed. Pour over salad and toss gently to coat.

58

Milk (Skim)   ☺ ☺ ☺

I consider milk the perfect Zone food because it contains a balanced ratio of protein to carbohydrates. An 8-ounce glass of skim milk provides you with a pretty good Zone snack, especially if you eat some high-quality fat at the same time. But since it contains carbohydrates, it can't be used to balance other forms of carbohydrate in your meal. Being the best source of calcium around, milk helps build healthy bones and teeth and helps maintain many of the basic functions of your body. Calcium wards off osteoporosis, and recent studies suggest that it may protect against high blood pressure and colon cancer as well.

Milk also gives you a healthy dose of vitamins A and D, riboflavin, and phosphorus. Drinking milk on a regular basis has been linked to lower stomach cancer rates in Japan and less lung cancer in international research surveys. Johns Hopkins researchers also found that smokers who drank milk were significantly less likely to develop chronic bronchitis compared with smokers who didn't drink milk. The researchers concluded that something in milk—possibly vitamin A—protected cells in the lung from damage by the tar in cigarettes.

Newer forms of skim milk have been concentrated to taste like the higher-fat forms but without the saturated fat. If you are lactose intolerant, I recommend trying lactose-free milk and other dairy products that are now prevalent in supermarkets as well as health food stores.

8 ounces of skim milk = 1 Zone Block

Strawberry Instant Breakfast

Serves 2

Block size

2 Protein	2 envelopes Knox Unflavored Gelatin
2 Protein	½ cup low-fat cottage cheese
2 Protein, 2 Carbohydrate	2 cups 1% milk
2 Protein, 2 Carbohydrate	1 cup plain low-fat yogurt
4 Carbohydrate	4 cups strawberries, sliced*
8 Fat	2⅔ teaspoons olive oil

Place all ingredients in blender to make instant breakfast. Blend until smooth. Pour into 2 large glasses, garnish with a strawberry, and serve.

*Fresh or frozen strawberries can be used. If using frozen strawberries, use whole or sliced berries without sugar or additives. If using fresh strawberries, use only those that are plump and have a solid color. Always store fresh strawberries covered in the refrigerator.

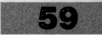

59

Protein Powder   ☺ ☺ ☺

Protein powders are a great way to supplement your Zone meals and snacks with instant protein. They're great for turning a fruit smoothie into a balanced Zone snack. Add protein powder to dips, oatmeal, and vegetable stir-fries to increase the protein-to-carbohydrate balance.

There are a variety of protein powders available. Isolated soy protein powder (the type I recommend is soy protein isolates) is the best kind because it has the least effect on your insulin levels. Soy protein powders don't taste as good as other protein powders, however, because of the presence of isoflavones. If you're not a vegan, you can try other protein powders. Some are made from deionized whey protein, a by-product of cheese production, which tends to taste better than other protein powders and also provides improved immunological stimulation compared with soy protein. Another kind is made from egg protein. These are better tasting but also produce greater insulin stimulation than soy protein powders. All of these powders can be stored at room temperature, ensuring easy access to protein to fortify any meal.

Did you know? The longest-living people in the world (the Okinawans) eat more than 100 grams per day of soy protein.

7 grams of protein powder = 1 Zone Block

Protein Power

Serves 1

Block size

3 Protein	20 grams protein powder
2 Carbohydrate	1 cup blueberries
1 Carbohydrate	1 cup strawberries
3 Fat	3 macadamia nuts
	4 ice cubes

Place all ingredients in a blender and blend at high speed until smooth, about 1 minute. Add a little water if smoothie is too thick. If you prefer, eat the nuts on the side.

Salmon   ☺ ☺ ☺

Salmon is one of the better-quality protein choices you can find. This is not so much because of its protein content (which is considerable) but for its rich supply of Omega-3 fatty acids. One 4-ounce serving gives you a whopping 2.1 grams of long-chain Omega-3 fatty acids, making it one of the best sources of Omega-3 you can find. These fatty acids help make "good" eicosanoids, which keep the blood from clotting abnormally and prevent excessive inflammation. This can help protect you from heart disease and other ravages of aging like wrinkles. Unfortunately, the higher levels of long-chain Omega-3 fats also mean higher levels of saturated fat, which brings down its overall protein rating slightly.

You can get a wide range of health benefits from a regular dose of Omega-3-rich salmon. These include:

- Reduced risk of atherosclerosis (plaque buildup in your arteries), blood clots, thrombosis, and arterial spasm
- Lower total cholesterol and triglycerides
- Improved blood sugar and insulin levels
- Possible reduction in the inflammation of arthritis and psoriasis
- Sharper mental functioning and improved concentration
- Reduced risk of mental illness such as schizophrenia and depression

Did you know? There are actually eight varieties of salmon that you can get in fish markets. Farm-raised Atlantic salmon is available all year but is thought to be less flavorful and possibly lower in Omega-3 fatty acids than the others. Of the seven types of Pacific salmon, chinook salmon is available from May to mid-June. Sockeye salmon (aka red) is available from mid-May to early August; it is the reddest variety and the highest in Omega-3s. Coho salmon (aka silver) is available fresh from July to September and is milder in flavor than the other varieties. Chum salmon and humpback salmon are often sold in cans or smoked. The other two varieties of Pacific Salmon are only available in Asia.

1½ ounces of salmon = 1 Zone Block

Poached Atlantic Salmon with Asparagus Coulis

Serves 6

Block size

                    1 bunch asparagus (peeled
                       and stems removed)
18 Protein, 18 Fat Six 4½-ounce Atlantic salmon
                       fillets (skin removed)

Court Bouillon:

1 quart purified water
1 cup dry white wine
1 small white onion, peeled
½ cup leek greens, diced
2 ribs celery
3 large bay leaves
1 teaspoon black peppercorns
½ cup parsley sprigs

Asparagus Coulis*:

                    3 large shallots, peeled and cut
                       in quarters
3 Carbohydrate   3 cups white leek, diced
                    ¾ cup + 1 cup chicken stock
3 Carbohydrate   36 asparagus spears
                    ¼ bunch sorrel
                    ¼ bunch watercress
                    Salt and white pepper, to taste

You may need additional asparagus for the coulis.

61

Dessert:

12 Carbohydrate	6 cups blueberries with a dollop of whipped cream (1 fruit cup per serving)

Peel and cut the woody stems from the asparagus. Reserve the peelings and stems. Blanch the asparagus in boiling water. Immediately cool and reserve for final presentation. Combine the ingredients for the court bouillon in a medium skillet or saucepan and simmer for 45 minutes.

For the coulis, simmer the shallots and white leek in ¾ cup of chicken stock for 20 minutes. Add the asparagus trimmings and the additional cup of chicken stock. Slowly braise the trimmings for 45 minutes or until all the greens are tender (retaining the brilliant green color). Stir in the sorrel and watercress and immediately remove from the stove. Strain off half the chicken stock and reserve. Puree the asparagus greens in a blender and strain through a fine sieve. The reserved cooking liquid may be used to correct the body of the coulis.

Now poach the salmon in the simmering court bouillon, 10 minutes per inch of thickness. Heat up the blanched asparagus in the reserved cooking liquid from the coulis recipe. Heat up the coulis (do not boil), check for the seasoning, and add salt and white pepper to taste. Place the coulis on a plate. Place the salmon on the coulis, and finish with two or three asparagus spears placed over the salmon.

Sardines   ☺ ☺ ☺

These small silvery fish pack more nutritional punch than you may realize. A 2-ounce serving of sardines (about four whole fish) serves up an amazing 400 percent of your vitamin B_{12} needs, almost 20 percent of your daily calcium requirement, and a moderate amount of long-chain Omega-3 fatty acids—all in just 100 calories. Plop some sardines on top of your salad and you've got a perfect Zone snack.

The Omega-3 fats in sardines protect the heart in numerous ways. Studies have found that eating just one to two servings of fish weekly cuts your risk of death from a heart attack. Omega-3 fats keep blood cells from sticking together, which reduces your risk of developing a blood clot that could lead to a heart attack or stroke. In addition, fish fat has been shown to lower high blood pressure, particularly if you have mild hypertension. Practically all sardines sold in the United States are canned, so look for them next to the canned tuna and clams in the supermarket.

Did you know? Sardines got their name because they were first harvested off the small Mediterranean island of Sardinia. They are actually a member of the herring family.

1½ ounces of sardines = 1 Zone Block

Mandarin Sardine Salad

Serves 1

Block size

½ Carbohydrate	1 cup celery, finely sliced
½ Carbohydrate	¾ cup red onion, finely sliced
1 Carbohydrate	½ cup Zoned French Dressing (see page 198)
½ Carbohydrate	½ peach, diced
1 Carbohydrate	⅓ cup mandarin oranges
	⅛ teaspoon turmeric
	1 tablespoon fresh mint, chopped
¼ Carbohydrate	1½ cups butterhead lettuce
¼ Carbohydrate	1½ cups romaine lettuce
4 Protein, 4 Fat	6½ pieces sardines, packed in soy oil, drained, skinless, boneless
	1 tablespoon fresh parsley, minced

In a salad bowl, combine celery, onion, Zoned French Dressing, peach, oranges, turmeric, and mint. Toss lightly. Arrange lettuce on a lunch plate, top with salad mixture, place sardines on top, and sprinkle parsley over all. Serve chilled.

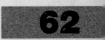

62

Zoned French Dressing

Four ¹/₂-cup servings

Block size

½ Carbohydrate
½ Carbohydrate
2 Carbohydrate
1 Carbohydrate

¾ cup onion, finely minced
¼ cup tomato puree
8 teaspoons cornstarch
¼ cup kidney beans, canned, rinsed, and minced
1¾ cups purified water
¼ cup cider vinegar
2 tablespoons balsamic vinegar
⅛ teaspoon Worcestershire sauce
1 teaspoon dried tarragon
1 teaspoon dried oregano
1 teaspoon dried parsley flakes
3 teaspoons garlic, minced
1 teaspoon dried basil
½ teaspoon chili powder
2 teaspoons paprika
1 teaspoon dried dill

Combine all ingredients in a small saucepan. (Mix cornstarch with a little cold water to dissolve it before adding to saucepan.) Heat dressing to a simmer, constantly stirring until mixture thickens. Let dressing cool for about 10 to 15 minutes, then place in a food processor and blend for 2 to 3 minutes until a smooth consistency forms. Transfer dressing mixture to a storage container, let cool, and refrigerate. This dressing may be refrigerated for up to 5 days or, if you prefer, may be frozen and defrosted for later use. Although the dressing is freeze-thaw stable, after it has been frozen and defrosted it may need to be stirred to reincorporate the small amount of moisture that forms on it during the freezing and thawing process.

Scallops   ☺ ☺ ☺

In terms of shellfish, scallops pack a powerful protein punch. Just 3½ ounces of scallops provide more than 23 grams of protein—compared with 12 grams of protein in clams and 14 in oysters. Scallops also provide a good source of vitamin B$_{12}$, which is necessary to prevent pernicious anemia. They also contain some magnesium and zinc.

A secretive animal that spends most of its short life hiding in underwater grasses, the scallop is a prized dinner entrée, especially in Florida, where the bay scallop is an important part of the marine ecosystem. Although bay scallops historically were a valuable seafood commodity, declining populations in many of Florida's coastal areas have prompted restrictions that now allow only recreational harvests.

Did you know? Since scallops are highly sensitive to changes in water quality, they are a good way to measure the health of an ecosystem. Just as coal miners once used canaries to detect low oxygen levels and the presence of dangerous gases in the mines, one type of scallop, called the bay scallop, provides an early warning system for scientists who monitor the quality of Florida's coastal waters.

1½ ounces of scallops = 1 Zone Block

Sautéed Scallops with Wine-Flavored Vegetables

Serves 1

Block size

4 Fat	1⅓ teaspoons olive oil, divided
4 Protein	6 ounces baby bay scallops
	½ teaspoon garlic, minced
	1 tablespoon fresh parsley, chopped
	½ teaspoon Worcestershire sauce
½ Carbohydrate	½ cup asparagus, chopped
2 Carbohydrate	2 cups artichoke hearts, chopped
½ Carbohydrate	1 cup red pepper, sliced
½ Carbohydrate	¼ cup Zoned French Dressing (see page 198)
½ Carbohydrate	¼ cup white wine
	Salt and pepper to taste

In a medium-size nonstick sauté pan, heat ⅔ teaspoon oil. Add scallops, garlic, parsley, and Worcestershire sauce. Sauté until scallops are cooked through. In a second nonstick sauté pan, add remaining oil, asparagus, artichokes, red pepper, and Zoned French Dressing. Cook until vegetables are crisp-tender. Add scallops and wine. Sauté an additional 3 to 5 minutes and spoon onto a serving dish. Salt and pepper to taste.

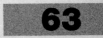

63

Sea Bass   ☺ ☺ ☺

If you're worried about the toxins in fish found in polluted waters, you can rest assured that sea bass is one of the safest fish around. It is caught offshore where waters are less polluted. Sea bass is also one of the healthiest fish you can eat. It is low in saturated fat, a good source of Omega-3 fatty acids, and contains moderate amounts of vitamins B_6 and B_{12} and magnesium.

When buying fresh sea bass, look for a fish that has clear, slightly bulging eyes, red slime-free gills, and shiny skin that isn't sticky. When buying fillets, look for flesh that is firm and elastic (pops back when pressed). Steer clear of sea bass that has a "fishy" smell. Truly fresh seafood has practically no fish odor.

Did you know? There are many different species of sea bass. The most fascinating is called the black sea bass, which can grow to incredible sizes. A world record 563-pound black sea bass was caught off the coast of Southern California in 1968. Although black sea bass can still be found around the islands of Southern California, their numbers are diminishing due to overfishing. There's now a moratorium on catching black sea bass until its population is replenished.

1½ ounces of sea bass = 1 Zone Block •

Broiled Sea Bass

Serves 1

Block size

3 Protein	4½ ounces sea bass
3 Fat	1 teaspoon olive oil
	Lemon or ginger slices
1 Carbohydrate	2 tomatoes, split, sprinkled with Parmesan cheese and broiled
1 Carbohydrate	1½ cups cooked green beans
1 Carbohydrate	½ cup grapes

Brush fish with olive oil. Place lemon or ginger slices on top. Broil 10 minutes per inch of thickness. Do not turn. Serve with tomatoes, green beans, and grapes.

64

Soybean Hamburger Crumbles ☺ ☺ ☺

This is a new version of soybean protein powder that resembles ground hamburger. This form has a much lower level of fat and therefore a better protein quality rating than boiled soybeans. I personally consider these soy hamburger crumbles to be the biggest breakthrough in soybean processing technology because they are so easy to use. This soybean product looks and tastes like real ground hamburger and can be used as a meat extender or substitute in casseroles, chili, or any other recipe that uses ground hamburger. It is incredibly easy to use because it can be taken directly from the refrigerator or freezer to the skillet and takes on spices and flavorings very readily.

Like other soy products, soy crumbles may confer certain health benefits: for example, the Japanese and Chinese have lower rates of heart disease and breast and prostate cancer than Americans, possibly because the Asian diets are rich in soy. Soy can help combat hot flashes and other menopausal symptoms. Researchers have also found that eating thirty or more grams of soy protein per day can reduce cholesterol levels. You can get about ten grams in four ounces of soybean hamburger crumbles.

⅓ cup of soy hamburger crumbles = 1 Zone Block

Sicilian Soy Sauce

Serves 1

Block size

3 Carbohydrate	1½ cups tomato sauce
4 Protein	1⅓ cups soybean hamburger crumbles (found in the freezer section, usually with the breakfast meats)
1 Carbohydrate	2 cups frozen sliced colored peppers
	Italian seasonings (e.g., garlic, onion, basil, oregano)
4 Fat	1⅓ teaspoons extra-virgin olive oil

Heat tomato sauce in medium saucepan. Add soy crumbles and peppers. Add fresh or dried Italian seasonings to taste. Cook over medium heat until done. Sprinkle with olive oil just before removing from heat.

65

Tuna   ☺ ☺ ☺

Tuna steak is the preferred form of tuna. Unfortunately, most of our experience probably comes from canned tuna, which has a slightly higher fat content (and lower Zone ranking). Nonetheless, grab a can opener and open a can of water-packed white-meat tuna. It's the easiest, most convenient way to get a reasonably good dose of long-chain Omega-3 fatty acids. One serving also has 40 percent of the RDA for vitamin B_{12} and is a good source of niacin. I can't emphasize enough how important long-chain Omega-3 fatty acids are for you. They can help reduce high cholesterol levels, normalize elevated blood pressure, prevent the formation of dangerous blood clots, and halt the growth of malignant tumors. They can also help boost your mental acuity and protect against mental illness such as depression and schizophrenia.

When mixing a tuna salad, hold the full-fat mayo, packed with saturated fat. Instead drizzle on some olive oil, Dijon mustard, and lemon juice.

Caveat: Don't go for the less expensive light tuna. You might save a few nickels, but you won't be getting as much Omega-3.

Did you know? Eating fish three times a week can significantly decrease your risk of heart disease. Researchers discovered the connection when they found that heart disease was exceptionally low among the Eskimos of Greenland, Japanese fishermen, and Native Americans of the Pacific Northwest. The one thing these three groups had in common? They all consumed fish rich in long-chain Omega-3 fatty acids as their main source of protein.

1 ounce of tuna steak or 1½ ounces of canned tuna = 1 Zone Block

Baked Tuna Steak
with Dill Sauce and Fruit

Serves 2

Block size

8 Fat	2⅔ teaspoons olive oil
8 Protein	8 ounces tuna steak
	2 teaspoons dried dill, divided
1 Protein, 1 Carbohydrate	½ cup plain low-fat yogurt
½ Carbohydrate	½ teaspoon sugar
	2 teaspoons white wine
½ Carbohydrate	2 teaspoons cornstarch
	Salt and pepper to taste
2 Carbohydrate	1 cup pineapple, cubed
1 Carbohydrate	½ cup blueberries
2 Carbohydrate	⅔ cup mandarin oranges
1 Carbohydrate	8 cherries, halved

Preheat oven to 375°F. Coat the bottom of a baking dish with oil, then place two 4-ounce pieces of tuna in bottom of baking dish. Sprinkle with 1 teaspoon of the dill, then tightly seal baking dish and bake for 25 to 30 minutes. While the tuna is baking, in a saucepan combine the yogurt, sugar, the rest of the dill, and the wine to make a dill sauce. Add a little water to the cornstarch and then add it to dill sauce. Stirring constantly, heat sauce through but do not bring to a boil. Add salt and pepper to taste. In a mixing bowl, combine pineapple, blueberries, orange sections, and cherries to make a fruit salad. Equally divide fruit salad between two lunch plates, then remove baking dish

66

from oven. Using a large spatula, scoop out tuna and place one piece of tuna on each plate. Pour an equal amount of dill sauce over each piece of tuna and serve immediately.

Turkey Breast, Skinless   ☺ ☺ ☺

You may think of turkey as a holiday food, but you shouldn't save it just for special occasions. Turkey is a great high-quality protein because it is so low in saturated fat. In fact, skinless turkey breast has the least fat and calories of any poultry choice. Even more good news: turkey is packed with nutrients, providing 50 percent of the RDA for folic acid in one 5-ounce serving. It's also a moderately good source of vitamins B_1 and B_6, zinc, and potassium.

Did you know? Turkey products, such as sausage, hot dogs, and ground turkey, may not be the nutritional dream you thought. If they are made with dark-meat turkey and ground turkey skin, they can contain as much saturated fat as beef versions. Be sure to read the label.

1 ounce of skinless turkey breast = 1 Zone Block

Oriental Turkey with Snow Peas

Serves 1

Block size

4 Fat	1⅓ teaspoons olive oil, divided
4 Protein	6 ounces lean ground turkey
½ Carbohydrate	5 cups alfalfa sprouts
1 Carbohydrate	2 cups bell pepper strips
½ Carbohydrate	¾ cup snow peas
½ Carbohydrate	¾ cup pearl onions, frozen
½ Carbohydrate	1½ cups broccoli florets
	1 teaspoon soy sauce
	1 teaspoon Worcestershire sauce
	1 tablespoon balsamic vinegar
1 Carbohydrate	¾ cup Zoned Espagnol (Brown) Sauce (see page 212)

In nonstick sauté pan, heat ⅔ teaspoon of the olive oil and cook the turkey (breaking it up as it cooks) and alfalfa sprouts. In second nonstick sauté pan, heat remaining olive oil and sauté peppers, snow peas, onions, broccoli, soy sauce, Worcestershire sauce, and vinegar. Cook until tender, then add Zoned Espagnol Sauce. Blend turkey mixture with vegetables and serve.

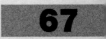

67

Zoned Espagnol (Brown) Sauce

Four ³/₄-cup servings

Block size

1 Carbohydrate	½ cup tomato puree
¼ Carbohydrate	¼ cup onion, finely diced
2¾ Carbohydrate	11 teaspoons cornstarch
	3 cups strong beef stock
	⅛ teaspoon Worcestershire sauce
	1 tablespoon red wine
	2 teaspoons garlic, chopped
	⅛ teaspoon dried oregano
	1 teaspoon dried parsley flakes
	Salt and pepper to taste

Combine all ingredients in a small saucepan. (Mix cornstarch with a little cold water to dissolve it before adding to saucepan.) Heat sauce to a simmer, constantly stirring with a whisk until mixture thickens. Transfer sauce mixture to a storage container, let cool, and refrigerate. This sauce may be refrigerated for up to 5 days or, if you prefer, frozen and defrosted for later use. Although the sauce is freeze-thaw stable, after sauce has been frozen and defrosted it may need to be stirred to reincorporate the small amount of moisture that forms on it during the freezing and thawing process.

Emu   ☺ ☺

Resembling an ostrich, an emu is a prehistoric bird that is thought to have roamed the outback of Australia for more than 80 million years. It provided the Australian Aborigines with food, clothing, shelter, and healing oils. Today emu has become a delicacy in the United States, providing a red meat similar in taste and appearance to very lean beef. In fact, emu has the lowest percentage of fat of any red meat, which gives it the highest ranking of any meat source on my Top 100 Zone Foods list. More importantly, most of the fat found in emu is the heart-healthy monounsaturated kind.

Emu can be purchased in a growing number of supermarkets or in gourmet meat markets. For more information, contact the American Emu Association at info@aea-emu.org.

Did you know? Emu oil is considered by many to be a healing potion. It has long been used as a topical agent to treat inflammation and burns.

1 ounce of emu = 1 Zone Block

Sautéed Emu with Spicy Apple Relish

Serves 1

Block size

4 Fat	1⅓ teaspoons olive oil
4 Protein	4 ounces emu fillet, diced, boneless, skinless
1 Carbohydrate	1½ cups red onion, chopped
	1 tablespoon cider vinegar
	½ teaspoon garlic, minced
	⅛ teaspoon sweet paprika
	Salt and pepper to taste
1 Carbohydrate	¾ cup Zoned Pepper Relish (see page 215)
2 Carbohydrate	1 Granny Smith apple, chopped
	¼ teaspoon chili powder

In a medium-size nonstick sauté pan, heat the oil. Add the emu, onion, vinegar, garlic, paprika, and salt and pepper. Sauté until cooked through. In a medium-size bowl combine Zoned Pepper Relish, apple, and chili powder. Spoon relish onto serving plate and top with emu.

68

Zoned Pepper Relish

Four ¾-cup servings

Block size

1½ Carbohydrate	3 cups frozen red and green bell pepper strips
½ Carbohydrate	¾ cup frozen onions, chopped
1 Carbohydrate	½ cup tomato puree
½ Carbohydrate	¾ cup tomato, chopped
½ Carbohydrate	2 teaspoons cornstarch
	¼ cup water
	1 tablespoon cider vinegar
	2 teaspoons pickling spice
	½ teaspoon lemon herb seasoning
	⅛ teaspoon celery salt

Combine all ingredients in a small saucepan. (Mix cornstarch with a little cold water to dissolve it before adding to saucepan.) Heat relish to a simmer, constantly stirring until mixture thickens. Simmer for 3 to 5 minutes until entire mixture is hot. Transfer relish mixture to a storage container, let cool, and refrigerate. This relish may be refrigerated for up to 5 days or, if you prefer, frozen and defrosted for later use. Although the relish is freeze-thaw stable, after it has been frozen and defrosted it may need to be stirred to reincorporate the small amount of moisture that forms on it during the freezing and thawing process.

Chicken Breast, Skinless   ☺ ☺

One of the healthiest forms of protein you can get, a 3-ounce serving of skinless chicken breast contains just 3 grams of fat, with a third of this amount coming from heart-healthy monounsaturated fat. What's more, chicken packs a hefty load of vitamin B$_6$—50 percent of the RDA in one 3-ounce serving—which helps lower levels of homocysteine (a substance that damages arteries). Chicken breast is also a good source of vitamin A.

Several research studies confirm the health benefits of chicken. In one, a group of people who ate chicken daily (in a typical Zone-size 3-ounce serving), as part of a diet low in saturated fat, experienced a drop in cholesterol levels. In the landmark DASH study, blood pressure dropped in participants who ate moderate amounts of chicken as part of a diet rich in fruits and vegetables.

Caveat: All parts of the chicken are not created equal. Avoid the skin and dark-meat portions, which are much higher in saturated fat and cholesterol.

Did you know? Chances are good that the chicken you buy is contaminated with a food-borne bacteria—usually campylobacter and more rarely salmonella. Cook raw chicken within two or three days of buying, and run chicken pieces under water before cooking to reduce bacteria levels. Chicken breast should be cooked thoroughly until the meat is white, not pink in the center. Use the leftovers within a day or two or freeze them.

1 ounce of skinless chicken breast = 1 Zone Block

Mediterranean-Style Chicken

Serves 2

Block size

8 Protein	8 ounces chicken tenderloins, flattened (or skinless chicken breast)
2 Fat	⅔ teaspoon olive oil
3 Carbohydrate	4½ cups tomato, diced
	8 garlic cloves, minced
	2 teaspoons dried basil
	1 teaspoon dried oregano
6 Fat	18 black olives, sliced
	4 tablespoons purified water
	2 tablespoons red wine
2 Carbohydrate	½ cup chickpeas
3 Carbohydrate	4½ cups eggplant, cut in ⅛-inch slices*

In a nonstick pan sauté chicken in olive oil until lightly browned. Add tomato, garlic, basil, oregano, olives, water, red wine, and chickpeas. Simmer, covered, for 10 minutes or until almost all the liquid evaporates. While the chicken is cooking, place eggplant in boiling salted water for 10 minutes, or until tender. On two dinner plates place a bed of cooked eggplant, then place the chicken-tomato mixture on top of the eggplant. Serve immediately.

When buying eggplants, look for those that are firm and have a deep purple color. The skin should have a glossy shine and be free of blemishes and discoloration.

69

Cottage Cheese (Low-Fat)   ☺ ☺

This is the one form of cheese that fits in well with the Zone Diet because of its low fat content relative to its protein content. Cottage cheese also plays a feature role in all my *Zone* books because it is such a versatile form of protein. You can mix it with fresh fruit or vegetables to have a Zone snack or stir it into a sauce or spread for your main course. According to the International Dairy Federation of America, cottage cheese consumption in the United States reached its peak of 1.1 billion pounds in 1972. Sales have been falling ever since, except for those of fat-free cottage cheese, which has seen its sales grow by double digits, increasing 14.6 percent in 1996.

Despite its dwindling popularity, cottage cheese deserves more attention. Some nationally sold brands are now fortified with calcium; others feature the same kinds of live bacteria found in yogurt, which may confer health benefits. Many organic brands of cottage cheese contain these live bacteria, and I highly recommend them. "Acidophilus and bifidus cultures" should appear on the list of ingredients on the label.

Did you know? Modern-day cottage cheese probably originated in ancient Rome. The Romans refined cheese-making techniques by experimenting with different curdling agents to come up with different varieties of cheese. Curd cheeses were a favorite at festivals, and cottage cheese was probably a top choice.

¼ cup of low-fat cottage cheese = 1 Zone Block

Mandarin Orange Cottage Cheese Scramble

Serves 1

Block size

4 Fat	1⅛ teaspoons olive oil
½ Carbohydrate	2 cups mushrooms, sliced
½ Carbohydrate	¾ cup onion, chopped
1 Carbohydrate	2 cups equal portions of red, yellow, and green peppers, cut in half and sliced
	1 tablespoon balsamic vinegar
	½ teaspoon Worcestershire sauce
	¼ teaspoon celery salt
	¼ teaspoon dried dill
3 Protein	¾ cup egg substitute
1 Carbohydrate	1½ cups snow peas, julienned
1 Protein	¼ cup low-fat cottage cheese
1 Carbohydrate	⅓ cup mandarin orange sections
	¼ teaspoon lemon herb seasoning

Heat oil in a medium-size nonstick sauté pan. Sauté mushrooms, onion, peppers, vinegar, Worcestershire sauce, celery salt, and dill. Cook until the vegetables are crisp-tender, about 5 to 7 minutes. Then pour in the egg substitute and snow peas. Cook, stirring, until set. Remove from heat and stir in cottage cheese and mandarin orange sections. Sprinkle on lemon herb seasoning and serve.

70

Shrimp   ☺ ☺

Shrimp can be part of a heart-healthy eating plan. In fact, when researchers from Rockefeller University in New York put volunteers on a diet of 11 ounces of shrimp a day—more than twice the recommended amount of cholesterol—the participants experienced no ill effects on their cholesterol levels and actually saw a 13 percent drop in their triglyceride levels. What's more, each serving of shrimp packs over 20 percent of your vitamin B_{12} needs, and can help protect your arteries from the damaging effects of the blood factor, homocysteine.

Use fresh shrimp within a day or two after purchasing, or freeze them for later use. Although there are many varieties of shrimp, the main difference is their size. Use small shrimp in fresh green salads or cold pasta salads. Use large shrimp for cold appetizers or baked in fajitas. Cook shrimp by stir-frying quickly in a nonstick pan, or grill them on spears.

Did you know? In the United States, shrimp is second only to tuna in popularity in the seafood category.

1½ ounces of shrimp = 1 Zone Block

Shrimp Scampi with Vegetables

Serves 1

Block size

3 Fat	1 teaspoon olive oil
1 Carbohydrate	12 asparagus spears, washed, woody bases discarded, and bias-sliced into 1-inch-long pieces
½ Carbohydrate	¾ cup yellow onions, peeled and finely chopped
½ Carbohydrate	1 medium green pepper, washed, cored, seeded, and roughly chopped
	2 cloves garlic, peeled and minced, or to taste
3 Protein	4½ ounces shrimp, shelled and deveined
	Optional: ¼ cup dry white wine
	1 to 2 teaspoons lemon juice, or to taste
	Optional: 2 lemon wedges
1 Carbohydrate	1 plum

In a large nonstick pan, heat oil over medium-high heat. Sauté asparagus, onions, green pepper, and garlic, stirring often until tender, about 10 minutes. Add shrimp, (optional) wine, and lemon juice. Lower heat to medium and cook 5 minutes, stirring often, until shrimp are pink. Place on plate, and if you wish, garnish with lemon wedges. Serve plum for dessert.

71

Soybean Imitation Meat Products ☺ ☺

Soybean imitation meat products include soy hamburgers, hot dogs, sausages, and deli meats. These are one step down from soy hamburger crumbles on the Zone protein quality ranking because they contain more fat. Like the soy hamburger crumbles, they are extremely versatile and make great additions to any meal.

Did you know? Although all soy imitation meat products are rich in protein, some—especially certain varieties of soy hamburgers—contain more carbohydrates than others. In fact, some contain more carbohydrates than protein! Be sure to read the labels and choose a brand that is lower in carbohydrates and contains less than 2 grams of fat per Zone Block of protein.

¾ soy hamburger patty, 1 soy sausage patty, or 3 slices of soy deli meats = 1 Zone Block

Vegetarian Burger

Serves 1

Block size

	Vegetable spray
2 Protein	1 soy burger patty
1 Protein	1 ounce reduced-fat cheese
.	Lettuce and tomato slice
	Optional: dill pickle wedge
2 Carbohydrate	1 slice rye bread
1 Carbohydrate	1 plum

Spray nonstick pan with vegetable spray. Cook soy burger 5 to 8 minutes on each side. (Check package instructions. Cooking directions vary from product to product.) Place cheese on cooked burger and top with lettuce, tomato, and pickle if desired. Serve on the rye bread with plum for dessert.

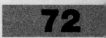

72

Soy Cheese   ☺ ☺

Soy cheese is made from soy milk. It has a creamy texture, making it easy to substitute for sour cream or cream cheese. It can be found in a variety of flavors in natural foods stores and supermarkets. Products made with soy cheese include soy pizza, and you can also make soy cheeseburgers. Soy cheeses are available as either hard cheese or cream cheese.

Soy cheese offers the same benefits as soy milk but has less carbohydrates. It is an excellent source of high-quality protein, B vitamins, and iron. Some brands of soy cheese are fortified with vitamins and minerals and are good sources of calcium and vitamins D and B_{12}. What's more, soy cheese is an excellent alternative for those who are lactose intolerant since it is free of the milk sugar, lactose.

Did you know? With soy yogurts made from soy cheese, you should read the label carefully, since many manufacturers add extra carbohydrates like sugar to improve the taste—just as they do for regular yogurt.

1 ounce of soy cheese = 1 Zone Block

Cheese and Veggie Melt

Serves 1

Block size

	3 to 4 tablespoons purified water (less for a gas range, more for electric)
	1 clove garlic, minced or pressed
	½ teaspoon dried basil, oregano, thyme, or combination
	Optional: ⅛ teaspoon ground black pepper
½ Carbohydrate	½ cup onion, cut in half-ring slices
½ Carbohydrate	1 cup red or yellow bell pepper, halved, seeded, cut in strips or 1-inch dice
⅓ Carbohydrate	1⅓ cups cremini or button mushrooms, thinly sliced
⅓ Carbohydrate	1 cup broccoli, cut in florets, stems peeled, cut thin
⅓ Carbohydrate	1⅓ cups cauliflower, cut into florets
1 Carbohydrate	½ cup carrots, cut in thin rounds or half-moons
4 Protein	4 ounces low-fat mozzarella, Colby, Monterey Jack, Muenster, or cheddar-style soy cheese, grated or cut in thin strips

73

| 4 Fat | 4 macadamia nuts or 12 almonds, raw or lightly toasted, coarsely chopped |
| 1 Carbohydrate | ½ cup grapes |

Add water, garlic, herbs, and spices to an 8- or 9-inch skillet with a lid. If cooking for two, use two small skillets or one 10- to 12-inch skillet; for four people, use a 12- to 13-inch skillet. Add vegetables to skillet in the order listed. Cover and bring to a boil. Reduce heat and simmer for about 4 to 6 minutes, or until almost tender. Remove lid from skillet; sprinkle nuts, then cheese over vegetables. Cover and simmer for 2 to 3 minutes or until cheese melts. (Or sprinkle on cheese, then cover and turn off heat.) Remove from heat. Use a spatula to transfer vegetables and cheese to a dinner plate. Serve immediately. Have grapes for dessert.

Tempeh   ☺ ☺

Tempeh, like soft tofu, makes the list in spite of being relatively rich in fat. However, that negative fact is overcome by the insulin-lowering effects of soy protein itself. A chunky, tender soybean cake that has a smoky or nutty flavor, tempeh is more easily digested than other traditional soy foods. It can be marinated and grilled or added to soups, casseroles, or chili. Since raw tempeh soaks up oil at an astonishing rate, your best bet is to brush each piece very lightly with oil and brown in a nonstick skillet. Tempeh contains the same heart-protective and cancer-preventive isoflavones as soybeans, and it offers its own unique benefits. Japanese scientists discovered that during the fermentation of tempeh, an anti-oxidant called HAA forms; this acts as a very strong protector against oxidative damage, the same type known to turn "bad" (LDL) cholesterol into an enemy of artery walls. Tempeh also packs a wallop of fiber and is a generous source of nutrients such as calcium, B vitamins, and iron.

Tempeh is typically sold in 8-ounce or 16-ounce vacuum-wrapped slabs, either refrigerated or frozen. You can find it in Asian or natural food stores. Don't be concerned if you notice any gray or blackish spots on the surface. This is simply the mold used to make tempeh, which can be cut away before the tempeh is cooked.

Caveat: Tempeh comes in many varieties depending on which ingredients are mixed with the soybeans. Pure soy tempeh has the strongest taste, while mixed-grain tempehs are a better choice for more delicate preparations and for newcomers to this tasty food. However, be careful to read the label of tempeh products because mixed-grain tempeh will contain higher amounts of carbohydrate that may make it unsuitable as a protein-rich source on the Zone Diet.

Did you know? In Indonesia, tempeh making is a household art that varies somewhat from home to home. Whole soybeans are usually mixed with a grain such as rice or millet. A starter—usually a piece of tempeh from a previous batch—is added to begin the fermentation process. In traditional home-based tempeh making, the mixture is wrapped in banana leaves and left to ferment for 18 to 24 hours.

1½ ounces of tempeh = 1 Zone Block

Tuscan Tempeh and Chickpea Casserole with Broccoli

Serves 1

Block size

Tempeh mixture:

	1 tablespoon tamari soy sauce
	2-inch piece kelp sea vegetable, scissor-cut into cubes
	1 bay leaf
	1 cup purified water
1 Carbohydrate, 4 Protein	6 ounces plain soy tempeh, cubed

Sauté mixture:

4 Fat	1⅛ teaspoons olive oil
¼ Carbohydrate	1 cup mushrooms, thinly sliced
½ Carbohydrate	½ cup onions, cut into thin half-ring slices
	1 clove garlic, minced or pressed
½ Carbohydrate	¾ cup chopped or diced tomato, with juices
¼ Carbohydrate	½ red or yellow bell pepper, cubed or cut in thin slices
	½ teaspoon each dried basil and oregano
	⅛ teaspoon ground red or black pepper

74

1 Carbohydrate	¼ cup cooked, drained chickpeas
½ Carbohydrate	2 cups broccoli, cut into florets, stems peeled and finely sliced
	Purified water for steaming

Combine tamari, kelp, bay leaf, and water in a 1- to 1½-quart saucepan. Add tempeh cubes. Cover, bring to a boil, then reduce heat and simmer without stirring for 30 minutes. Remove lid and simmer away liquid. Tempeh is ready to use now. Discard bay leaf. Chop kelp. Add oil to 10-inch skillet and heat, adding mushrooms and onions. Stir until softened, reducing heat as needed to prevent scorching. Add garlic, tomato, bell pepper, herbs, spices, cooked tempeh, kelp pieces, and chickpeas. Bring to a boil, reduce heat to medium-low, cover, and simmer for about 20 minutes, until tender and liquid is reduced. Mixture should resemble a thick stew. When tempeh casserole is almost done, place broccoli in a vegetable steamer over boiling water in a medium-size saucepan. Cover and steam for about 5 to 6 minutes or until broccoli is vibrant green and crisp-tender, not soggy or gray. Immediately transfer broccoli to a serving plate. Top with tempeh casserole. Serve.

Variation

After cooking tempeh, you may set one-fourth aside (one Zone Protein Block) for tomorrow. Grate 1 ounce nonfat mozzarella cheese and sprinkle over tempeh casserole just before serving.

Tofu   ☺   ☺

Also known as soybean curd, tofu is a soft cheeselike food made by curdling fresh hot soy milk. Depending on how much liquid is extracted from the curd, the tofu is labeled as soft, medium, firm, or extra-firm. The firmer the tofu, the more protein it contains relative to carbohydrate and the less fat. This is why extra-firm tofu is a better Zone choice than soft tofu. Besides being a good source of protein, tofu supplies plenty of B vitamins and iron. Tofu may also give you a hefty dose of calcium when the curdling agent used to make it is calcium salt. Adding to this nutritional arsenal, tofu provides plenty of isoflavones, disease-fighting substances that may help ward off heart disease and cancer.

Fresh Chinese-style organic tofu is readily available in vacuum-packed 1-pound blocks in refrigerated tubs. Sealed, refrigerated tofu is a better choice than the small squares of tofu that you'll find soaking in water at room temperature in Asian grocery stores. These are open to air and possible contamination and usually aren't made from organic soybeans.

When purchasing tofu, note the expiration date. Once you've opened the container, refrigerate any leftovers in water in a tightly sealed container. Change the water every day or so, and the tofu will remain fresh for about five days. Tofu is often called the chicken of the vegetable kingdom, since it has a mild taste that readily takes on a wide variety of flavors. Use firm tofu in stir-fries, kebobs, or any dish that requires tofu to hold its shape. Use soft tofu (a creamy kind) to make dips, dressings, vegetable purees, and smoothies.

Did you know? Tofu was first used in China around 200 B.C. Although the discovery of the process for making tofu is lost to the ages, Chinese legend has it that the first batch of tofu was created by accident. A Chinese cook added the curdling agent, *nigari*, to flavor a batch of pureed cooked soybeans; the *nigari* produced the curd that we know today as tofu.

3 ounces of extra-firm tofu, 4 ounces of firm tofu, or 6 ounces of soft tofu = 1 Zone Block

Ginger-Scallion Tofu Stir-Fry

Serves 1

Block size

½ Carbohydrate	2 cups mushrooms, sliced
	1 tablespoon lite soy sauce
	⅛ cup of vegetable stock (see page 71)
	1 tablespoon fresh ginger, minced
	1½ cloves garlic, minced
1 Carbohydrate	1½ cups tomatoes, chopped
4 Protein	8 ounces extra-firm tofu, thinly sliced
4 Fat	1⅓ teaspoons canola oil
2 Carbohydrate	3 cups snow peas, thawed if frozen
½ Carbohydrate	1½ cups scallions, cut into 1-inch pieces

Combine mushrooms, soy sauce, vegetable stock, ginger, garlic, tomatoes, and tofu in a bowl and marinate 30 minutes. Heat oil in a heavy skillet or wok over medium-high heat. Add tofu mixture and stir-fry 3 to 4 minutes. Add snow peas and scallions and stir-fry 3 to 4 minutes or until snow peas are bright green.

75

Trout   ☺   ☺

Trout is a good source of Omega-3 fatty acids. The benefits of Omega-3 fatty acids are numerous. They can help lower cholesterol and triglyceride levels, reducing your risk of heart disease. They may also lower blood pressure, and prevent the formation of clots that can cause heart attacks and strokes. They may prevent the growth of cancerous tumors and can help prevent depression and schizophrenia.

In 4 ounces of trout, you get 1.1 grams of long-chain Omega-3 fatty acids as well as a healthy dose of vitamin B_{12} and more than 10 percent of the RDA for iron, all of which can help prevent anemia.

Caveat: Trout is found in lakes and streams, many of which have become dumping grounds for polluters. I recommend buying trout that has been raised on a fish farm.

Did you know? Several studies have found that eating 8 ounces of fish a day can relieve the painful symptoms of rheumatoid arthritis. This positive change is not permanent, however; when the research subjects stopped eating fish, their symptoms could quickly return.

1½ ounces of trout = 1 Zone Block

Kodiak Trout with Green Beans

Serves 1

Block size

	Canola oil cooking spray
	½ teaspoon Worcestershire sauce
	⅛ teaspoon celery salt
4 Protein, 4 Fat	4½ ounces raw wild rainbow trout fillet
2 Carbohydrate	3 cups green beans, cut into 2-inch pieces
1 Carbohydrate	1½ cups onion, chopped
	½ teaspoon garlic, minced
	2 teaspoons cider vinegar
	⅛ teaspoon nutmeg
	⅛ teaspoon cinnamon
	⅛ teaspoon lemon herb seasoning
	⅛ teaspoon ground double superfine mustard
	½ teaspoon soy sauce
	Salt and pepper to taste
	1 teaspoon fresh parsley, minced
	1 lemon wedge
1 Carbohydrate	1 peach for dessert

Spray canola oil into a medium-size nonstick sauté pan. Heat. Blend in Worcestershire sauce and celery salt. Add trout fillet and sauté until cooked through and browned on both sides. Set aside. Spray a second nonstick sauté

76

pan. Heat oil and add green beans, onion, garlic, vinegar, nutmeg, cinnamon, lemon herb seasoning, mustard, soy sauce, and salt and pepper. Cook until beans are crisp-tender. Place beans and fish on serving plate. Sprinkle with parsley and place lemon wedge to one side. Serve immediately.

Yogurt ☺ ☺

Like milk and soy milk, natural yogurt is a perfect Zone food, providing the right ratio of protein to carbohydrate. But be careful to read the label, since most fruit-flavored yogurts contain a huge amount of carbohydrates that can send you right out of the Zone. Add some high-quality fat to it for additional flavor. A 1-cup serving of nonfat plain yogurt provides a hefty 40 percent of your calcium needs. Calcium is essential for good bone health and also appears to play a role in preventing high blood pressure. Plain yogurt is also rich in the mineral potassium, which plays a role in maintaining blood pressure.

Yogurt may additionally provide some benefit to your cholesterol levels. One study of volunteers ages 55 to 70 found that those who ate a daily serving of yogurt kept their total cholesterol and "bad" (LDL) cholesterol levels steady while they rose in a group of volunteers who did not eat yogurt. You've no doubt heard that yogurt may help destroy harmful microorganisms in the digestive tract and may even help extend longevity. These health claims are unproven, but I still endorse yogurt wholeheartedly. You can, of course, eat yogurt as a snack by itself, but you can also try it in salad dressings, sandwich spreads, dips, and smoothies.

Did you know? Americans consume approximately 5 pounds of yogurt yearly per person—five times more than in 1970.

6 ounces of yogurt = 1 Protein Block

"Egg Nog" Yogurt with Fruit

Serves 1 to 4

Block size

2 Protein, 2 Carbohydrate	1 cup plain low-fat yogurt
2 Protein	⅔ ounce unflavored or unsweetened vanilla soy protein powder (14 grams protein)
	½ to 1 teaspoon pure vanilla extract (nonalcohol, glycerine base)
	Scant ⅛ teaspoon turmeric powder
	⅛ teaspoon ground nutmeg
	⅛ to ¼ teaspoon stevia extract powder
4 Fat	1⅓ teaspoons almond oil or 12 almonds, raw or lightly toasted, chopped coarsely
1 Carbohydrate	⅓ banana, cut in thin slices*
1 Carbohydrate	1 peach, halved, pitted, sliced*

Place yogurt in small bowl or 1-quart Pyrex measuring cup. Add protein powder, vanilla, turmeric, nutmeg, and stevia. Stir well with a large spoon, scraping the sides as needed to incorporate all of the seasonings.

If slicing fruit in advance of serving, either drizzle it with lemon juice or place it in the bottom of serving containers, then top with "Egg Nog" Yogurt.

77

Taste. Add ⅛ teaspoon additional stevia if a sweeter taste is desired. Stir in almond oil or sprinkle nuts on top. Top with sliced fruit just before serving. Serve immediately or pour into one container (for a breakfast) or four containers (to yield four snacks). Cover and refrigerate.

Variations

Replace banana with 2 dates, finely chopped.

Replace 1 peach with ½ cup blueberries. If desired, also replace ⅓ banana with ½ cup blueberries.

Soy Milk   ☺   ☺

Soy milk is made from ground soybeans that are sim-
mered in water and pressed to extract a nutrient-rich
beige liquid. It is an excellent source of high-quality
protein, B vitamins, and iron. Some brands of soy milk
are fortified with vitamins and minerals and are good
sources of calcium, vitamin D, and vitamin B$_{12}$. Soy milk
is free of the milk sugar, lactose, and is a good choice for
people who are lactose intolerant. Also, it is a good alternative for those who are allergic to cow's milk.

With its unique nutty flavor and rich nutrition, soy
milk can be used in a variety of ways—virtually any
way you would use cow's milk. You can use it to make
smoothies or pour it into your morning oatmeal. Soy
milk is sold in boxes that can be stored at room temperature until they are opened, but be sure to use them
before the expiration date on the package. Opened containers will last for a week to 10 days in the refrigerator. Soy milk is also sold as a powder, which must be
mixed with water.

Caveat: Keep in mind that soy milk, like skim milk and
boiled soybeans, contains carbohydrates, which means
that it can't be used as a pure protein source for making
Zone meals. As a snack, it's OK. Furthermore, when
shopping for soy milk, check the labels and compare
brands, as manufacturers may add a wide range of
sweeteners and other ingredients, often extra carbohydrates, to enhance its appeal to the American palate.
These extra carbohydrates eliminate the natural balance
of protein to carbohydrates found in soy products.

Did you know? In China and Japan, soy milk is sold by street vendors and in cafés. It is served hot or cold and is often sweetened or flavored with soy sauce, onion, and vegetables to produce a spicy soup.

8 ounces of soy milk = 1 Protein Block

Zoned Cocoa-Banana Cherry Freeze

Serves 1 to 8

Block size

¾ Protein, ¾ Carbohydrate	½ cup soy milk, chilled
4 Fat	4 teaspoons unsweetened almond or macadamia nut butter
3¼ Protein	1 ounce + 1 tablespoon unflavored or unsweetened vanilla soy protein powder (23 grams protein)
¼ Carbohydrate	1 heaping tablespoon unsweetened cocoa powder
	1 teaspoon pure vanilla extract (nonalcohol, glycerine base)
	Optional: ⅛ to ¼ teaspoon stevia extract powder or 2 to 4 drops stevia extract liquid
	Optional: 1 tablespoon apple fiber powder
1 Carbohydrate	⅓ ripe medium banana, peeled, sliced, and frozen (about ⅓ cup)
2 Carbohydrate	1½ cups frozen unsweetened cherries
	Optional: 3 to 4 ice cubes (from purified water)

78

Pour soy milk into a blender. Add nut butter, protein powder, unsweetened cocoa, vanilla, and (optional) stevia. Add apple fiber powder, if desired, for added thickness and blood sugar control. Cover and blend until smooth. Stop and scrape down the sides with a spatula. With motor running, add frozen fruit through the top feeder. When blended, add (optional) ice cubes one or two at a time, blending on the ice-crushing setting until desired thickness. Stop and start blender, pushing the pulse button repeatedly until ice is completely crushed and mixture is smooth and thick. Try a spoonful. Add more stevia if a sweeter taste is desired. Pour into four custard cups or dessert dishes and serve immediately. Or pour into four to eight small paper cups, then freeze until firm, about 3 hours. If frozen solid, remove from freezer 10 to 15 minutes before serving, or as needed to soften to an ice cream texture. Alternatively, pour into a tall fountain glass to serve one person for breakfast.

Beef Tenderloin, Well-Trimmed   ☺

On the Zone Diet, you might think you can never indulge in a piece of meat, but that's wrong. It's true that some cuts of meat give you hefty amounts of saturated fat, which is bad for your heart and your waistline. Beef tenderloin (which is cut into filet mignon), however, is a great source of protein because it is lean—but *only* if you have removed all the separable fat. If you do so, then a 3-ounce serving of lean tenderloin (the average meal-size serving for a woman on the Zone) contains just 170 calories and 8 grams of total fat. Surprisingly, beef tenderloin is richer in monounsaturated fat than saturated fat.

You might also be surprised to discover that beef is loaded with important vitamins and minerals. Lean beef is rich in the B vitamins such as B_{12}, riboflavin, B_6, and niacin. A 3-ounce serving also provides about 20 percent of the RDA for iron, nearly 40 percent of the RDA for zinc, and a considerable amount of potassium. All of these vital nutrients can help prevent disabling diseases. Iron and B_{12} can help prevent anemia. (The iron in beef is more easily absorbed by the body than the iron found in vegetable and grain sources.) B_{12} deficiency in older adults can cause memory loss, confusion, and mood changes. Zinc and B_6 help keep your immune system humming.

Did you know? Beef consumption has fallen by more than 25 percent since 1976. Even so, the average American consumes more than 60 pounds a year, and the amount of beef we're consuming has begun to rise again. The current fat content of beef is 27 percent less than it was in the early 1980s, largely because of consumer demands for leaner meat.

1 ounce of well-trimmed beef tenderloin = 1 Zone Block

Spiced Pepper Steak

Serves 1

Block size

4 Fat	1⅓ teaspoons olive oil
	⅛ teaspoon garlic powder
4 Protein	4 ounces lean beef, thinly sliced
	⅛ teaspoon Worcestershire sauce
	2 tablespoons cider vinegar
1 Carbohydrate	4 cups mushrooms, sliced
1 Carbohydrate	2 cups red and green pepper strips
1 Carbohydrate	1½ cups onion, sliced
1 Carbohydrate	½ cup Zoned Herb Dressing (see page 68)

Heat oil in medium-size nonstick sauté pan. Sprinkle garlic powder onto beef. Sauté beef until cooked. Deglaze pan with Worcestershire sauce and vinegar. Add vegetables and stir-fry 5 to 7 minutes. Combine beef and vegetables in medium-size bowl and add Zoned Herb Dressing. Toss to coat. Spoon onto plate and serve.

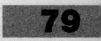
79

Pork Tenderloin, Well-Trimmed   ☺

In the early 1990s, pork became a verboten food because of its reputation as a high-fat food. Many cuts of pork, however, are relatively lean if you remove all the separable fat. If you do, then calorie for calorie, they are an excellent source of vitamins, minerals, and protein. A 3-ounce well-trimmed broiled loin chop contains just 165 calories and 8 grams of fat, which compares pretty well against a 3-ounce leg of lamb, which has 13 grams of fat (mostly the heart-damaging saturated kind). What's more, pork is a great source of vitamin A and iron and supplies a moderate amount of B vitamins, zinc, and folic acid. All of these vitamins and minerals are essential for your body's proper functioning.

Caveat: It's best to eat cured pork in only moderate amounts because it contains nitrites, chemicals that combine with others in your digestive tract to form cancer-causing compounds. Also, make sure your pork is well cooked, since undercooked pork can contain parasites.

1 ounce of well-trimmed pork tenderloin = 1 Zone Block

Pork Tenderloin with Apple Compote

Serves 1

Block size

4 Fat	1⅓ teaspoons olive oil, divided
4 Protein	4 ounces pork tenderloin
2 Carbohydrate	1 Granny Smith apple, cored and chopped
1 Carbohydrate	⅓ cup unsweetened applesauce
	2 tablespoons cider vinegar
	⅛ teaspoon celery salt
	⅛ teaspoon cinnamon
	2 tablespoons lemon-and-lime-flavored water
	¼ teaspoon lemon herb seasoning
1 Carbohydrate	4 cups mushrooms, sliced

Heat ⅔ teaspoon of oil in a medium-size nonstick sauté pan. Sauté pork loin until cooked through and lightly browned. Add apple, applesauce, vinegar, celery salt, cinnamon, flavored water, and lemon herb seasoning. Simmer for 3 to 5 minutes. In second nonstick sauté pan, heat remaining oil. Add mushrooms and cook for 3 to 5 minutes. Spoon mushrooms onto a serving plate. Top with pork mixture and serve.

80

Soybeans (Boiled)   ☺

Referred to as the "wonder bean" or *ta-tou,* which in Chinese means "greater bean," soybeans are indeed a wondrous food to behold because they are the only beans that contain more protein than carbohydrate. A cup of cooked beans packs about 25 percent of your daily requirement for fiber and folate along with a hefty 29 grams of soy protein, which is one of the best proteins you can eat. Why? Soy protein has less of an effect on your insulin levels than does animal protein. So with a greater amount of insulin control, it can significantly enhance the beneficial effects of the Zone even more than high-quality animal protein. In fact, I devoted an entire book, called *The Soy Zone,* to adapting the Zone Diet by using soy protein in place of animal protein.

An analysis of 38 clinical studies published in *The New England Journal of Medicine* in 1995 found that consuming an average of 50 grams of soy per day lowered cholesterol levels by 9 percent. This level of cholesterol reduction should lead to a 20 percent reduction in heart disease risk. Other studies have linked soy consumption to a decreased risk of breast cancer, prostate cancer, and osteoporosis.

Boiled soybeans are actually a mixture of carbohydrate, protein, and fat, thus making a perfect Zone snack all on their own. It's almost as if Mother Nature favored the Zone ratio when she created soybeans.

Use boiled soybeans as you would any other bean, in salads, casseroles, soups, or as a snack on their own.

Caveat: Boiled soybeans contain a significant amount of carbohydrate, which prevents them from balancing off other forms of carbohydrates.

⅓ cup of cooked soybeans = 1 Protein Block

Baked Soybean Casserole

Serves 4

Block size

	2 quarts water
4 Carbohydrate, 6 Protein, 6 Fat	2 cups cooked soybeans, drained
1 Carbohydrate	1 cup tomato sauce
½ Carbohydrate	¾ cup yellow onion, peeled and finely diced
	2 cloves garlic, peeled and minced
	1 teaspoon dry mustard
	2 teaspoons chili powder
	1 teaspoon ground black pepper
½ Carbohydrate	½ tablespoon dark molasses
4 Fat	12 almonds, slivered

Preheat oven to 300°F. In a large Dutch oven or oven-proof pot, combine 2 quarts of water with all ingredients except almonds. Bake for 3 hours, stirring occasionally. If casserole becomes dry during cooking, add water in small increments. Allow to cool for 10 minutes before serving. Sprinkle slivered almonds on top just before serving.

FATS

Macadamia Nuts   ☺ ☺ ☺

This is the champion of Zone fats. They have the highest fat ranking since they are very rich in monounsaturated fats, with very low levels of saturated and Omega-6 fats. They also provide moderate amounts of calcium. A 3½-ounce serving provides 40 mg of calcium.

A native of northeastern Australia, the macadamia nut is now also grown commercially in Hawaii. Notoriously difficult to extract from their shells, they are expensive but have a delicious creamy flavor and crunchy texture. If you want to maximize the monounsaturated fat in your diet, consider munching on some macadamia nuts, since they are small controlled balls of a great Zone fat that will do wonders for your hormonal system.

Did you know? According to an ancient aboriginal legend, macadamia nuts were first discovered when a tribesman named Baphal fell and hurt his foot while standing guard over a mountain to protect his people. Although he was unable to collect food for himself, a cockatoo flew out, gathered nuts, and scattered them near him. When Baphal's people finally came to rescue him, they saw him munching on strange nuts. They called them "Baphal's nuts."

1 macadamia nut = 1 Zone Block

Fruit Salad with Macadamia Nuts

Serves 1

Block size

½ Carbohydrate	5 cups romaine
1 Carbohydrate	¾ cup Zoned Pepper Relish (see page 215)
4 Protein	1 cup low-fat cottage cheese
1 Carbohydrate	½ Granny Smith apple, cored and chopped
1 Carbohydrate	⅓ cup mandarin orange sections
½ Carbohydrate	1½ teaspoons raisins
	Salt and pepper to taste
4 Fat	4 macadamia nuts, chopped

Form a bed of romaine on a serving plate. Top with Zoned Pepper Relish. In a medium bowl, combine cheese, apple, orange sections, raisins, and salt and pepper. Mix well. Mound cheese on top of lettuce and sprinkle with nuts.

Olive Oil ☺ ☺ ☺

Olive oil is one of the true superstars of Zone fats. It is one of the reasons that people who live in Mediterranean countries like Greece, Italy, Spain, and southern France have much lower rates of heart disease than Americans. While Americans wolf down burgers and fries loaded with saturated fat, people who live near the Mediterranean eat olive oil as their main source of fat. More than 70 percent of olive oil is monounsaturated fat, the heart-healthy kind that lowers blood cholesterol levels and appears to protect artery walls from oxidation damage. Olive oil is also very low in Omega-6 fatty acids, which can accelerate heart disease and cancer by the overproduction of "bad" eicosanoids.

Use olive oil as you would any other fat on the Zone Diet—in moderate amounts. A little goes a long way in terms of taste. Use light olive oil when you don't want such a strong flavor and extra-virgin oil when you want a stronger taste in salads or as a marinade for tofu, chicken, or fish.

Did you know? Olive oil has been a health potion around the Mediterranean for 4,000 years. Ramses II, who ruled Egypt between 1300 and 1200 B.C., was rumored to have gulped down olive oil for every complaint.

⅔ teaspoon of olive oil = 1 Zone Block

Olive Oil Mushroom Artichoke Deluxe

Serves 1

Block size

4 Fat	1⅛ teaspoons olive oil
1 Carbohydrate	1½ cups onions, chopped
2 Carbohydrate	2 cups artichoke hearts, diced
4 Protein	4 ounces beef tenderloin
1 Carbohydrate	1 cup Zoned Mushroom Sauce (see page 255)

In a nonstick sauté pan, add oil, onion, artichoke hearts, and beef. Cook until beef is done and vegetables are tender. Add Zoned Mushroom Sauce and heat through. Place mixture on a large dinner plate and serve immediately.

83

Zoned Mushroom Sauce

Serves 4

Block size

1½ Carbohydrate	6 cups mushrooms, sliced
2½ Carbohydrate	10 teaspoons cornstarch
	3 cups strong beef stock
	⅛ teaspoon Worcestershire sauce
	1 tablespoon red wine
	⅛ teaspoon chili powder
	½ teaspoon garlic, chopped
	1 tablespoon dried parsley flakes
	Salt and pepper to taste

Combine all ingredients in a small saucepan. (Mix cornstarch with a little cold water to dissolve it before adding to saucepan.) Heat sauce to a simmer, constantly stirring until mixture thickens. Transfer sauce mixture to a storage container, let cool, and refrigerate. This sauce may be refrigerated for up to 5 days or, if you prefer, the sauce may be frozen and defrosted for later use. Although it is freeze-thaw stable, after it has been frozen and defrosted it may need to be stirred to reincorporate the small amount of moisture that forms on it during the freezing and thawing process.

Almonds   ☺ ☺

In a nutshell, almonds are great for your heart. Seems contradictory that fat is good for the heart, but it's true. A landmark study of 26,000 members of the Seventh-Day Adventist Church found that those who ate almonds at least six times a week had an average lifespan of seven years longer than the general population and a substantially reduced risk of heart attack. The reason is simple: almonds are rich in monounsaturated fats, the good kind that reduce cholesterol and thus protect against heart disease. Almonds also contain vitamin E, which thins the blood, helping to prevent blood clots that can cause heart attacks and strokes.

Almonds are a sliver above other nuts because they are an excellent source of nondairy calcium. An ounce of almonds provides about 10 percent of the RDA for this mineral.

Did you know? Historians generally agree that almonds and dates, both mentioned in the Bible, were among the earliest cultivated foods. In classical times, the Romans distributed sugared almonds as gifts to great men at public and private events.

3 almonds = 1 Zone Block

Almond Cottage Cheese and Fruit

Serves 4

Block size

4 Protein	1 cup low-fat cottage cheese
1 Carbohydrate	¾ cup cantaloupe, cubed
1 Carbohydrate	½ cup honeydew melon, cubed
1 Carbohydrate	½ cup canned peaches, cubed
1 Carbohydrate	½ cup pineapple, cubed
4 Fat	4 teaspoons slivered almonds

Place ¼ cup cottage cheese in a mound in the center of four serving dishes. Surround the cottage cheese with fruit cubes and sprinkle with almonds.

84

Avocados   ☺ ☺

Contrary to what you might think, avocados are a fruit, not a vegetable. But I consider avocados to be a fat, since they contain primarily fat. One medium-size (8-ounce) California avocado contains a whopping 30 grams of fat. This fat is mostly the monounsaturated kind, which does not elevate blood cholesterol levels as saturated fat does and, in fact, actually increases "good" (HDL) cholesterol.

When served as part of a Zone meal, an avocado contributes a number of important nutrients. A few slices of avocado provide a hefty serving of potassium and folate along with a small amount of iron, magnesium, and vitamins A, C, E, and B₆. How many other fats—like butter and margarine—can make the same claim? Avocados should be served raw since they have a bitter taste when cooked.

Did you know? The avocado is popularly known as the alligator pear because of the shape and rough skin of its most common variety. Unlike most fruits, avocados start to ripen only after being cut from the tree. The avocado came from Persia. It has been popular in South America, Central America, and Mexico for centuries. The ancient Aztecs left evidence that the avocado was in their diet, as did the Mayans and the Incas. Jamaicans also dined on avocados in the seventeenth century.

1 tablespoon of avocado = 1 Zone Block

Basic Guacamole

Block size

10 Fat

1 ripe avocado
Lemon juice
Salt and freshly ground white
    pepper

Buy a nice ripe avocado, free of bruises. To ripen an avocado, place it in a paper bag for a day or two. Cut the avocado in half lengthwise, and remove the peel and pit. In a glass bowl, mash the avocado with the lemon juice, salt, and pepper until it is smooth. Cover and refrigerate it until ready to use. (Optional: Add some chopped tomato and onion.)

85

Canola Oil   ☺ ☺

This new all-purpose cooking oil has one of the lowest levels of saturated fat combined with a high level of monounsaturated fat. However, it has higher levels of Omega-6 fatty acids, which makes it one step down from olive oil.

Canola oil is virtually tasteless, so it's great to use for baking and in foods where you're not after that Italian flair. Like any Zone fat, a little canola oil goes a long way. Consider using a pump spray when cooking with canola oil, since you can easily pour on too much.

Did you know? Canola oil is a genetically engineered oil, which has become the national crop of Canada as well as a significant oilseed crop for the United States. It was originally derived from rapeseed oil and engineered to reduce the amounts of erucic acid.

⅔ teaspoon of canola oil = 1 Zone Block

Hong Kong Burger

Serves 1

Block size

4 Fat	1⅓ teaspoons canola oil
4 Protein	1⅓ cups soybean hamburger crumbles (found in the freezer section, usually with the breakfast meats)
	¼ teaspoon fresh ginger, grated
	1 clove garlic, minced
½ Carbohydrate	1½ cups cooked broccoli
½ Carbohydrate	2 cups raw sliced mushrooms
2 Carbohydrate	⅔ cup canned sliced water chestnuts
	1 tablespoon lime juice
	2 teaspoons Asian fish sauce
	⅛ teaspoon crushed red pepper
	2 red lettuce leaves
1 Carbohydrate	1 cup red onion, thinly sliced
	¼ scallion, chopped
	1 tablespoon fresh cilantro, chopped

Heat canola oil in a heavy nonstick skillet over medium-high heat. Sauté soy crumbles, ginger, garlic, broccoli, mushrooms, and water chestnuts for 10 minutes, stirring often, until mixture is warmed throughout. Stir in lime juice, fish sauce, and red pepper. Bring to a boil and

86

cook 1 to 2 minutes, until liquid has evaporated by half. Arrange lettuce on a serving dish. Mound hot soy mixture in center. Garnish with red onion, scallion, and cilantro.

Cashews   ☺ ☺

The cashew is very rich in heart-healthy monounsaturated fats, similar to the almond. It's very versatile and tastes great in chicken and beef dishes or sprinkled on salads. Monounsaturated fats offer more than just heart benefits. A study from Sweden found that a high intake of monounsaturated fats reduced a woman's risk of breast cancer by 45 percent compared with a diet high in Omega-6 and saturated fat.

A 3½ ounce serving of cashews provides 60 mcg of vitamin A and 4 mg of iron. Native to America but now grown extensively in India and East Africa, the cashew can withstand drier conditions than most other nuts. Related to mangos and pistachios, the cashew nut grows in a curious way on the tree, hanging below a fleshy, applelike fruit.

Did you know? Cashew shells contain urushiol, the same irritating oil that's found on poison ivy leaves. Heating inactivates the urushiol, so you can safely eat toasted cashews. However, you should never eat the raw nuts.

3 cashews = 1 Zone Block

Melon-Cashew Medley

Serves 1

Block size

1 Carbohydrate	½ cup melon balls
4 Protein	1 cup low-fat cottage cheese
1 Carbohydrate	¾ cup peach chunks
1 Carbohydrate	¾ cup cherries
1 Carbohydrate	⅛ cup mandarin orange sections
4 Fat	4 teaspoons crushed cashews

Cut two small melons in half to form four melon bowls. If necessary, cut the ends of the melons so that the melon bowls will sit on a plate without moving. Using a melon baller, remove the flesh by scooping out the melon. Leave a thin border wall inside the melon bowls. Mound cottage cheese in the center of each melon shell. In a mixing bowl combine remaining fruits, then divide equally and spoon over cottage cheese in melon bowls. Garnish with cashews and serve.

Peanuts ☺

Despite their name, peanuts aren't really nuts at all but legumes like lentils and black beans. And the same heart-protective chemical found in red wine, resveratrol, is also found in the red skin of peanuts. Since peanuts contain 14 grams of fat per 1 ounce serving, I consider them a fat—although they do contain some protein as well. Peanuts contain lower amounts of monounsaturated fat than olives or almonds, which is why they have a lower Zone fat quality ranking. A serving of peanuts also supplies about 20 percent of the RDA for vitamin E, the vitamin responsible for protecting your arteries from damaging LDL cholesterol. They also contain a good amount of folate.

With all these nutrients, it's no wonder that regular peanut munching has health benefits that can be measured in research studies. One study of more than 30,000 women done at Loma Linda University in California found that women who ate peanuts and other nuts four times a week or more had half the risk of heart attacks compared with women who ate peanuts less than once a week.

Did you know? Scientists from the University of Florida have invented a new, "healthier" peanut that contains 80 percent of the heart-healthy oleic fatty acid, compared with about 50 percent in regular peanuts. This change also gives peanuts a longer shelf life and supposedly enhances their taste. You've probably already eaten this "new and improved" peanut without even knowing it.

6 peanuts = 1 Zone Block

Stir-Fry Tofu with Peppers and Peanuts

Serves 1

Block size

1 Fat	6 peanuts
3 Fat	1 teaspoon peanut oil
4 Protein	8 ounces extra-firm tofu, cubed
	1 clove garlic, pressed
	½ teaspoon fresh grated ginger
1 Carbohydrate	3 turnip tops, washed and coarsely chopped
½ Carbohydrate	1⅓ tablespoons rice wine or sherry vinegar
½ Carbohydrate	1 teaspoon pure maple syrup
	1 tablespoon tamari or shoyu sauce
	2 teaspoons arrowroot dissolved in 2 teaspoons purified water
	Optional: ½ teaspoon chili or Tabasco sauce
½ Carbohydrate	1 small onion, diced
1 Carbohydrate	1 small green bell pepper, diced
	1 small red bell pepper, diced
½ Carbohydrate	12 mushrooms, sliced
	2 scallions, sliced

Roast peanuts in toaster oven or under broiler for 3 to 5 minutes, turning twice. Set aside. Combine peanut oil and tofu in skillet and sauté over high heat. After 5 minutes, add garlic and ginger. Sauté another 3 minutes and remove from skillet. Rinse and steam turnip tops in steamer basket over boiling water, or boil in small amount of water with no basket, until tender, about 10 minutes. Set aside with lid half off. Mix rice wine vinegar, maple syrup, tamari, arrowroot, and (optional) Tabasco in a small bowl. Combine onion, peppers, and mushrooms in a skillet and sauté 5 minutes on medium-high heat. Add water if necessary and stir regularly. Stir up sauce in bowl and add to skillet. Stir until thickened. Add tofu and heat through, about 3 minutes. Serve over bed of warm turnip tops. Top with peanuts and scallions.

SPICES AND CONDIMENTS

Garlic

Garlic tops the list of foods being investigated by the National Cancer Institute for its disease-fighting properties. Where to begin? How about with the more than 500 major studies that have been performed on garlic in recent years. From this vast body of research, scientists know that allicin, a chemical that forms when garlic is crushed, reduces cholesterol levels and lowers blood pressure. It also seems to reduce the ability of platelets to form blood clots, thus reducing the risk of heart disease and strokes.

Another compound, called diallyl sulfide (DAS), has been shown to inactivate potent cancer-causing substances in animal studies. It also suppresses the growth of tumors. Garlic compounds also stimulate the formation of glutathione, an amino acid that is a potent antioxidant. Scientists still don't know whether garlic confers more health benefits when it is crushed and cooked or chopped and added raw to foods. After reviewing the scientific research, I believe that any form of fresh garlic is effective in lowering cholesterol and improving circulation.

Did you know? Although we've only recently focused on garlic as a medicinal food, garlic was appreciated as a healing food in ancient times. The Egyptians worshipped it and placed clay models of garlic bulbs in the tomb of Tutankhamen. Hippocrates used garlic bulbs to treat cervical cancer, and monks chewed on garlic to protect themselves against the plague in the Middle Ages.

Lamb with Garlic Cheese and Vegetable "Pasta"

Serves 4

Block size

12 Protein	12 ounces lean loin lamb chops
6 Fat	2 teaspoons olive oil
	1 cup dry red wine
	3 garlic cloves, baked
6 Fat	1 tablespoon unsalted butter
	Optional: salt and pepper
	1 ounce goat cheese or Rondelé light cheese
	Chopped parsley from 6 sprigs; reserve 4 sprigs for garnish

Preheat oven or toaster to 350°F. Remove outer skin from garlic cloves. Arrange garlic cloves in small baking dish. Dot with olive oil. Cover dish with aluminum foil and bake for one hour. Uncover, and bake fifteen minutes longer.

Trim the fat off the chops, and skewer to keep them together to cook more evenly. In a heavy skillet (enameled, cast iron or heavy stainless steel), heat the oil until very hot. Cook the chops in two batches. Brown the first side, turn over, and salt the seared side. Cook the other side, until the chops are medium rare. Remove to a plate. Cook the remaining chops and remove to a plate.

Pour off the fat and add the red wine. Cook over

89

medium heat until the wine has slowly reduced by half. Press the baked garlic cloves through a small strainer, and add them to the skillet with the butter. Whisk for a moment to emulsify the butter into the sauce.

Taste it and add salt and pepper if you wish. Serve two chops per person with some sauce, and add the juice from the plate. Top with goat or Rondelé cheese. Sprinkle with finely chopped parsley and garnish with parsley sprigs. Serve with Vegetable "Pasta" (see recipe on page 271).

Vegetable "Pasta"

Serves 4

Block size

3 Carbohydrate	2 to 3 medium-size carrots
3 Carbohydrate	4 medium-size yellow squash
3 Carbohydrate	4 medium-size zucchini
3 Carbohydrate	¾ cup cooked white beans
3 Fat	1 teaspoon butter or olive oil
	Salt
	Freshly ground pepper
	¼ cup chopped basil
	¼ cup chopped parsley
	Fresh herbs such as basil or
	dried herbs

Wash and peel the carrots. Wash the zucchini and the squash. With a vegetable peeler, slice the zucchini and squash into long strips. Shred the carrots with a potato peeler into long shreds, and then discard the center core of the carrot or reserve for soup. Set aside until ready to cook.

Over medium heat in a large, heavy stainless-steel skillet or a wok, heat the butter or oil. Add the shreds. Cook the carrot first, for 2 to 3 minutes, then add the squash, zucchini, and beans and toss frequently, cooking for 3 to 4 minutes. (Note: Olive oil allows you to heat the skillet to a higher temperature.) Add salt, pepper, and chopped herbs. Serve immediately with lamb chops.

Basil

Along with its robust flavor, basil provides potent anti-oxidants called monoterpenes that may help protect against heart disease and cancer. Basil may also help stabilize blood sugar levels in people with adult-onset diabetes. Researchers in India gave basil leaf preparations to diabetic patients and found that fasting blood glucose levels dropped by more than 17 percent. Italian researchers report that eating basil, as well as parsley and rosemary, may reduce lung cancer risk. In other research, the growth of cancers such as liver tumors was stunted in animals that were fed basil leaves.

Did you know? The classical name *basilicum*, from which the name *basil* is derived, means "royal" or "princely." The Hindus consider basil to be a sacred plant, referring to it as "holy basil," and believe that it is an incarnation of a goddess. Hindus worship basil beginning each year in May when the seeds are sown and continue nurturing the seedlings for a period of three months while the plant grows. In the fall, a festival is held in honor of basil.

Tomato Basil Salad

Serves 1

Block size

1 Carbohydrate	10 cups romaine lettuce, chopped
½ Carbohydrate	¼ cup salsa*
½ Carbohydrate	¼ cup Zoned Herb Dressing (see page 68)
1 Carbohydrate	¼ cup chickpeas, rinsed and finely chopped
	1 tablespoon fresh parsley, chopped
4 Fat	1⅓ teaspoons olive oil
	1 tablespoon red wine vinegar
	2 tablespoons fresh basil, chopped
	1 teaspoon garlic, minced
	¼ teaspoon chili powder
1 Carbohydrate	1½ cups tomatoes, sliced
4 Protein	4 ounces skim milk mozzarella cheese, shredded

In a medium-size bowl, combine lettuce, salsa, and Zoned Herb Dressing, then form into a bed on a serving plate. In a second bowl, blend chickpeas, parsley, oil, vinegar, basil, garlic, and chili powder. Alternate slices of tomato and shredded mozzarella on lettuce bed. Pour chickpea dressing over tomatoes and serve.

We used a medium-heat salsa. Use whatever strength you prefer.

90

Alfalfa Sprouts

Well-known biologist Frank Bouer called alfalfa "the great healer" because the delicate sprouts contain sparse amounts of unwanted calories and fat and abundant amounts of good-for-you fiber. For centuries, healers have used alfalfa in herbal medicine, but modern-day scientists are just beginning to recognize its healing properties. In fact, alfalfa sprouts are among the richest sources of anti-oxidative capacity per gram of carbohydrate.

Alfalfa is also a good source of vitamin K, which helps your blood clot to prevent hemorrhaging and also helps your body retain calcium. As if all these health benefits weren't enough, alfalfa sprouts also contain phytoestrogens, which are plant chemicals that act like the hormone estrogen. Menopausal women suffering from hot flashes and mood swings may be able to counteract their symptoms with alfalfa.

Caveat: Children, the elderly, and people with compromised immune systems should not eat raw alfalfa sprouts, recommends the Food and Drug Administration. They should eat sprouts only if they have been cooked thoroughly. The agency issued this advisory after outbreaks of food-borne illness occurred in people who ate sprouts contaminated with the bacteria *E. coli*.

Did you know? The alfalfa plant is extremely fast growing and has massive roots for its size, extending as deep as 250 feet into the ground to draw up needed nutrients in the soil.

10 cups of alfalfa sprouts = 1 Carbohydrate Block

Omelette with Sprouts and Herbs

Serves 1

Block size

4 Fat	1⅓ teaspoons olive oil
½ Carbohydrate	¾ cup onion, chopped
½ Carbohydrate	1 cup red and green bell peppers, chopped
½ Carbohydrate	2 cups mushrooms, sliced
	¼ teaspoon garlic, minced
	⅛ teaspoon dried oregano
	⅛ teaspoon dill
	⅛ teaspoon chili powder
	⅛ teaspoon dried parsley
	⅛ teaspoon Worcestershire sauce
	⅛ teaspoon cilantro
	Dash of lemon herb seasoning
4 Protein	1 cup egg substitute
½ Carbohydrate	5 cups alfalfa sprouts
1 Carbohydrate	⅓ cup mandarin orange sections
1 Carbohydrate	½ cup salsa*

In a nonstick sauté pan, heat oil over medium-high heat. In a medium-size bowl, combine the onion, bell peppers, and mushrooms. Add garlic, oregano, dill, chili powder, parsley, Worcestershire sauce, cilantro, and

*Salsa comes with different levels of heat. Choose one that best fits your tastes.

91

lemon herb seasoning. Spoon vegetable/herb mixture into pan and sauté for 3 minutes, until vegetables soften and herbs are heated. Pour egg substitute into pan, stir to distribute vegetables, and cook until almost set. Sprinkle sprouts onto half of omelette and fold over. Remove to serving plate. Decorate with orange sections, and top omelette with salsa.

Chili Peppers

Chili peppers became hot (no pun intended) a few years ago when research came out showing that eating chilies could help keep you thin by speeding up your metabolism. After eating hot chilies, you tend to sweat—to help you reduce internal body temperature (this is a real plus in warm climates). Chilies are rich in a compound called capsaicin, which gives them their biting sting but, paradoxically, also relieves pain. This is because capsaicin drains cells of a chemical called substance P, which sends pain signals out through nerve cells to the brain. The rush you get from a chili pepper also triggers the release of feel-good hormones called endorphins, which can cause you to feel slightly euphoric.

Chili peppers benefit the body as well as the mind. One pepper will give you a full day's supply of beta-carotene and nearly twice the RDA for vitamin C. In animal studies, chilies have been shown to reduce cholesterol levels by lowering LDL and triglycerides. Even more good news: contrary to popular belief, chili peppers will not cause ulcers and will not promote stomach distress or harm an otherwise normal stomach. But they should not be eaten by those who have existing ulcers or stomach problems.

Did you know? The botanical name of chili peppers, *Capsicum frutescens,* is derived from the Greek word for "bite," *kapto,* and bite they do. When Columbus took his first bite of a chili, he thought he had discovered a new source for pepper, a highly valued spice. Chilis aren't related to peppercorns, but the name stuck anyway.

Vegetarian Chili with Peppers

Serves 1

Block size

3 Protein	1 cup soy protein crumbles
3 Fat	1 teaspoon olive oil
	Onions, chopped, to taste
	Garlic, to taste
1 Carbohydrate	1 cup chopped green peppers
	2 cups red peppers
	Pepper, to taste
	Mushrooms, to taste, chopped
1 Carbohydrate	1½ cups chopped, stewed tomatoes with liquid
2 Carbohydrate	½ cups kidney beans, drained and rinsed
	Chili powder, to taste
1 Protein, 1 Fat	1 ounce reduced-fat cheese, shredded

Sauté the crumbles in the oil with the chopped onion, garlic, peppers, and mushrooms. Add tomatoes, kidney beans, and chili powder. Simmer until beans are tender. Top with shredded cheese.

92

Cinnamon

I consider cinnamon to be almost a magical spice. When sprinkled on foods, it imparts a sweetness that can almost be mistaken for sugar—but without the damaging effects on insulin. What's more, cinnamon provides a host of health benefits. Richard Anderson of the U.S. Department of Agriculture's Human Nutrition Center, found that certain spices actually stimulate the efficiency of insulin, so you require less of the hormone to process sugar. Anderson's tests on animals found that sage and oregano double insulin activity, turmeric and cloves triple activity, and cinnamon is the most potent of all. Although no studies have been done in humans, Anderson reports that many diabetics have told him that adding 1 teaspoon of cinnamon to their diets each day had a beneficial effect on their blood sugar level. I am a true believer because I sprinkle a liberal amount of cinnamon on my slow-cooked oatmeal every time I eat it.

Adding to cinnamon's virtues, a recent study from George Washington University found that cinnamon may also play a role in lowering blood pressure.

Did you know? Cinnamon has been popular since ancient times, starting with the Egyptians who imported it from China in 2000 B.C. The Romans believed cinnamon was sacred, and the emperor Nero burned a year's supply of the spice at the funeral for his wife. A major motive for world exploration in the fifteenth and sixteenth centuries: the search for cinnamon.

Apple-Cinnamon Raisin Omelette

Serves 2

Block size

4 Carbohydrate	2 red Delicious apples, cored and sliced
2 Carbohydrate	2 tablespoons raisins
	½ cup purified water
2 Protein	2 envelopes Knox Unflavored Gelatin
2 Carbohydrate	⅔ cup applesauce
8 Fat	2⅔ teaspoons olive oil, divided
	½ teaspoon plus ⅛ teaspoon cinnamon
6 Protein	8 egg whites plus 2 whole eggs*
	⅛ teaspoon turmeric

In a medium-size nonstick sauté pan, place apples, raisins, and water. Simmer mixture over medium heat for 3 to 4 minutes, until apples soften slightly. In a mixing bowl, add gelatin, applesauce, ⅔ teaspoon oil, and ½ teaspoon cinnamon. Add applesauce mixture to apple-raisin mixture and mix well, simmering an additional 3 to 4 minutes. Place apple-applesauce mixture aside and keep warm. In a mixing bowl, whip egg whites, whole eggs, and turmeric together. Heat 1 teaspoon oil in a second sauté pan. Pour half the egg mixture into the sauté pan and cook until egg sets and an omelette

*Eggs used in this recipe are sized as large.

93

forms. As the omelette is cooking, lightly sprinkle with a dash (⅛ teaspoon) of cinnamon. When omelette is cooked, place half the filling on omelette and fold over. Remove to serving plate and serve immediately. Repeat process to make second omelette.

Curry Powder

Although sold as a single spice, curry powder is actually a combination of spices: turmeric (which gives curry its golden color), cinnamon, garlic, ginger, cardamom, coriander, and cumin, as well as other spices. These make for a powerful combination that provides a one-two punch against disease. Some of the compounds in the spices are potent anti-oxidants that protect normal cells from damage by cancer-causing free radicals. Other compounds have an antibiotic effect that can help thwart bacteria that can cause food poisoning.

Research has found that curry spices can also lower cholesterol and prevent the formation of blood clots. These spices can also reduce inflammation, which can relieve the aches and pains associated with arthritis. A recent study sponsored by the USDA shows that turmeric boosts the ability of insulin to metabolize glucose, which may help control diabetes.

Did you know? For centuries, curry powder has been used by Indian healers to aid digestion. Before refrigeration, many curry spices were used to prevent food from going rancid. Back in those times, no one knew why the spices worked. Now we know that the spices are powerful agents against bacteria and other germs that can spoil food.

Thai Green Fish Curry

Serves 2

Block size

8 Fat	2⅔ teaspoons olive oil
1 Carbohydrate	1½ cups snow peas, whole
1 Carbohydrate	1½ cups onion, chopped
	4 garlic cloves, minced
1 Carbohydrate	1½ cups hot peppers, in rings
	4 teaspoons vinegar
6 Protein	9 ounces fresh fish fillets, cut in slivers
2 Protein, 2 Carbohydrate	1 cup plain low-fat yogurt
	1½ cups water
	1 teaspoon turmeric
	4 teaspoons hot curry powder
	Salt and pepper to taste
1 Carbohydrate	4 teaspoons cornstarch
2 Carbohydrate	½ cup chickpeas, drained

In a nonstick sauté pan, add oil, snow peas, onion, garlic, hot peppers, and vinegar. Cook until vegetables are tender, then add fish, yogurt, water, chickpeas, and remaining spices. Cover sauté pan and poach fish in vegetable liquid until cooked through. When the fish is cooked, mix the cornstarch with a little water and add to sauté pan. Bring mixture to a boil, then simmer for an additional 5 to 10 minutes. Divide between two soup bowls and serve.

94

Ginger

Ginger is a multipurpose spice both for cooking and healing purposes. The Chinese have used it to zip up their cuisine since 600 B.C., and the Europeans relied on ginger to drown out the bad taste of often spoiled meat during the Middle Ages. Ginger is also a great healer. It combats nausea caused by motion sickness or morning sickness during pregnancy and may help relieve stomach upset.

Researchers have been studying ginger's other health benefits, namely its ability to reduce the risk of heart disease. Danish investigator K. C. Srivastava claims that ginger is a more potent blood thinner than either garlic or onion—two well-known blood thinners. He gave heart disease patients a single 2-teaspoon dose of powdered ginger and then took a blood sample to measure its degree of "stickiness," an indication of how easily the blood would clot. The ginger significantly reduced the ability of the blood to clot, working in a similar way as aspirin. By the same token, researchers from India found that ginger "brings down drastically" the blood cholesterol levels of rats over the long term. The spice was shown to offset the cholesterol-raising effects of a high-fat diet.

I wouldn't recommend trying to down 2 teaspoons of ginger in one sitting, which would be hard on your taste buds. Do try to use ginger liberally, however; mix it in salad dressings, stir it into steamed vegetables, and sprinkle it on grilled fish. Add a piece of gingerroot to a cup of hot tea.

Did you know? Ginger is recognized internationally as a healing spice, but different countries use it for entirely different medical purposes. Asian physicians prescribe fresh gingerroot for vomiting, coughing, stomach upset, and fever; Africans drink gingerroot as an aphrodisiac; whereas women in New Guinea eat the dried root as a contraceptive. In India, children are given fresh ginger tea for whooping cough.

Stir-Fry Chicken with Ginger Vegetables

Serves 1

Block size

4 Fat	1⅛ teaspoons olive oil, divided
4 Protein	4 ounces chicken tenderloin in ½-inch cubes
	3 teaspoons fresh gingerroot, minced, divided
	2 teaspoons garlic, minced, divided
½ Carbohydrate	2 cups mushrooms, sliced
1 Carbohydrate	2 cups cabbage, shredded
½ Carbohydrate	¾ cup snow peas
1 Carbohydrate	⅛ cup water chestnuts
½ Carbohydrate	1½ cups scallions in ¼-inch pieces
½ Carbohydrate	2 cups cauliflower florets
	1 tablespoon soy sauce
	½ cup chicken broth

Heat ⅔ teaspoon oil in a medium-size nonstick sauté pan. Add chicken, 1 teaspoon ginger, and 1 teaspoon garlic. Stir-fry until chicken is cooked and garlic is lightly browned. In a second nonstick sauté pan heat remaining oil and stir in mushrooms. Cook for 2 minutes. Add cabbage, snow peas, water chestnuts, scallions, cauliflower, soy sauce, broth, and remaining ginger and garlic. Stir-fry until cabbage and cauliflower are tender. Place vegetables on serving dish and top with chicken.

95

Lemons

Ideal for flavoring everything from fish to fruits to vegetables, lemons are among the most widely used citrus fruits. I put them on my condiment list because not many of us can stomach eating a single lemon in one sitting. Like other citrus fruits, lemons are a great source of vitamin C; the juice from a single lemon has more than 50 percent of the RDA. Vitamin C is a potent antioxidant that helps prevent cancer and heart disease and reduces your chances of getting an infection. Lemons are also a good source of limonene, a citrus oil that has been shown to thwart cancerous tumors in animals. As if this weren't enough, lemons are rich in terpenes, substances that control the production of cholesterol.

To get the most juice from a lemon, let it sit in warm water for a few minutes before squeezing. Another tip: if your recipe calls for grated lemon zest, be sure to wash the peel thoroughly before grating since it often contains pesticide residues.

Did you know? Lemons date back 2,500 years to Asia. In the twelfth century, the Arabs brought lemons to Spain and Africa. According to Spanish historian Las Casas, Christopher Columbus brought lemon seeds with him from the Canary Islands on his second voyage to America.

Lemon Meringue

Serves 4

Block size

Lemon filling:

2 Carbohydrate	⅔ cup apple juice
½ Carbohydrate	Juice of ½ lemon
	½ tablespoon agar flakes
	1 teaspoon lemon extract (nonalcohol, glycerine base)
½ Carbohydrate	1 teaspoon sugar
	1 teaspoon arrowroot powder dissolved in 1 teaspoon water
2 Protein	4 ounces extra-firm tofu
	2 teaspoons olive oil

Meringue:

2 Protein	4 egg whites, at room temperature
	¼ teaspoon cream of tartar
1 Carbohydrate	2 teaspoons sugar

Preheat oven to 400°F. Combine apple and lemon juice, agar, lemon extract, olive oil, and sugar in a small saucepan and simmer until agar dissolves, about 5 minutes. Remove from heat and add arrowroot, stirring constantly until it disappears. Pour sauce into blender, add tofu, and blend until smooth. Pour into small ovenproof dish or miniature pie plate. Put aside to set.

Beat egg whites with cream of tartar until stiff. Add sugar and beat a moment longer. Pile the meringue onto lemon filling and bake for 5 to 7 minutes until golden.

Miso

The Japanese have used miso for centuries as an intense spice to flavor clear soups and other traditional dishes. Miso is made from crushed soybeans inoculated with mold to trigger fermentation along with a lot of salt and a grain such as rice or barley. This paste is then aged for a few years before it's ready for use. Miso is packed with the heart-protecting power of soybeans. It contains compounds called isoflavones, which have been shown to lower cholesterol levels and reduce heart disease risk. Miso also supplies you with fiber, iron, and zinc, along with folic acid, which helps protect artery walls from damage that can lead to heart disease.

You can find miso at your local supermarket or Asian food store. It should be refrigerated after opening. Since miso has such a high sodium content (over 5,000 mg in ½ cup) and an intense flavor, it will serve you best as a condiment to season your vegetables and soups.

Caveat: If you have salt-sensitive high blood pressure, you're better off avoiding miso and using natto, a similar soybean paste that has virtually no sodium.

Did you know? Miso is a daily part of the Japanese diet; a typical Japanese meal contains one vegetable dish with rice and a cup of miso soup. The classic Japanese word for miso soup is *omiotsuke*: it is a combination of three words of respect in Japanese (*o, mi,* and *o*). No other food gets such high reverence in the Japanese language.

Chunky Miso Soup

Serves 1

Block size

2 Carbohydrate	1 tablespoon barley
	4 cups purified water or vegetable stock (see page 71)
4 Fat	1⅓ teaspoons toasted sesame oil
¼ Carbohydrate	1 small onion, chopped
¼ Carbohydrate	2 medium stalks celery, chopped
¼ Carbohydrate	6 medium white mushrooms, sliced
	2 medium shiitake mushrooms, stems removed and sliced
¼ Carbohydrate	¼ medium cabbage, shredded
	2 thin slices fresh ginger, peeled
	Optional: 6 to 8 green or wax beans
1 Carbohydrate	¼ cup kidney beans, cooked
	4 tablespoons red barley miso paste
4 Protein	8 ounces extra-firm tofu
	1 scallion, sliced

Combine barley and water or stock in large pot, bring to a boil, and simmer covered for 20 minutes. In a sauté pan, add sesame oil and sauté onion and celery over medium heat for 3 to 4 minutes. Add mushrooms and cabbage and sauté 2 to 3 minutes more. Add the sauté, ginger, and

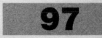

97

(optional) green beans to barley broth and simmer covered for 20 minutes. When ready to serve, remove 1 cup of broth from pot and stir into miso paste until smooth. Return broth and miso paste to the pot, remove from heat, and stir gently. Do not cook miso! Cooking miso can destroy its beneficial properties. Add tofu and let stand for 2 to 3 minutes. Stir once before serving in soup bowls. Garnish with scallion slices.

Parsley

You may think of parsley as little more than a garnish on your plate at restaurants. I want you to banish this thought. Parsley can't afford to be overlooked for what it is: an herb stocked full of nutrients. A handful of parsley (about 10 sprigs) provides 10 percent of the RDA for beta-carotene and 15 percent for vitamin C. What's more, parsley is a member of the umbelliferous vegetable family, which the National Cancer Institute has recognized for its cancer-fighting potential. Some of the potent chemicals in parsley include:

- Polyacetylenes, which halt the production of eicosanoids that may promote cancer
- Coumarins, which help prevent blood clotting, reducing your risk of arterial blockages that can lead to heart attacks
- Flavonoids, some of which are anti-oxidants that neutralize dangerous free radicals, others of which deactivate hormones that trigger tumor growth
- Monoterpenes, anti-oxidants that help fight cancer and reduce cholesterol

Not bad for a bit of plate dressing!

Did you know? Historical records show that parsley was fed to chariot horses in the time of the Roman Empire because it was believed that it would make them run faster. Parsley was also sold for centuries as a multipurpose cure for any ailment. Those health claims may not have panned out, but parsley is a great breath freshener. Parsley tea works very well: steep 10 sprigs of parsley in a cup of hot water for 10 minutes and flavor with a little honey or lemon.

Gourmet Rock Cornish Hen à l'Orange

Serves 2

Block size

8 Protein	1 Rock Cornish game hen, roughly 2 pounds (half of weight is in bone)
8 Fat	2⅔ teaspoons olive oil, divided
1 Carbohydrate	3 cups mushrooms, diced fine
	4 garlic cloves, minced
	2 teaspoons parsley
2 Carbohydrate	3 cups onion, diced fine
	½ teaspoon paprika, divided
	½ cup chicken stock
	⅛ teaspoon white wine
	½ teaspoon orange extract (nonalcohol, glycerine base)
2 Carbohydrate	⅔ cup mandarin orange sections
½ Carbohydrate	2 teaspoons cornstarch
1 Carbohydrate	3 cups broccoli spears
1½ Carbohydrate	3 cups red bell pepper, diced
	Salt and pepper to taste

Preheat oven to 400°F. Using a large sharp knife, slice Rock Cornish hen in half along the backbone. Remove tail and skin and discard, along with gizzards. Set hen aside. In a sauté pan, add ⅔ teaspoon oil, mushrooms, garlic, parsley, and onion. Cook until mixture is translucent (about 10 minutes). (This mixture is known as a *duxell*. A duxell consists of finely cooked vegetables

98

used to stuff another item.) When the duxell is cooked, set aside to cool. Sprinkle each Rock Cornish hen half with ¼ teaspoon paprika and rub it with remaining oil. Form two mounds of duxell in a casserole dish, place hen halves on top, and gently press them into the duxell. Tightly seal the casserole with aluminum foil and bake for 45 minutes. While the hen halves are cooking, combine stock, wine, orange extract, and orange sections in a small saucepan. Add cornstarch to a little water and then stir into saucepan. Cook over medium heat until the liquid thickens to form a sauce. In another saucepan, add broccoli and bell pepper with enough water to cover. Cook until tender. Remove casserole dish from oven and drain off any juices. Using a large spatula, scoop out duxell and hen halves as one piece and place on two dinner plates. Pour orange sauce over each hen half and add an equal amount of broccoli and bell pepper to each plate. Salt and pepper to taste. Serve immediately.

Salsa

It's a great flavoring and a fun dip, but salsa as a wonder food? Actually it is, in more ways than one. This mixture of cooked tomatoes, peppers, and onions is packed full of anti-oxidants like vitamin C and cancer-preventive phytochemicals. In fact, research has shown that the phytochemical lycopene, found in tomatoes, is actually more potent in cooked tomato products like salsa. One study found that men who ate cooked tomato products like tomato sauce, ketchup, and salsa several times a week had a reduced incidence of prostate cancer. The chili peppers in salsa give you a healthy dose of beta-carotene, another anti-oxidant.

Did you know? Salsa has overtaken ketchup as America's most popular condiment.

Chips and Salsa Snack

Serves 1

Block size

1 Carbohydrate

½ ounce baked tortilla chips

1 Fat

1 tablespoon pureed avocado

1 tablespoon salsa*

1 Protein

1 ounce cheddar cheese, fat-free, shredded

Place tortilla chips on snack plate. Blend avocado with salsa and pour over tortilla chips, then sprinkle with shredded cheese and serve.

Salsa comes with different levels of heat. Choose one that best fits your taste.

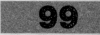

99

Sesame Seeds

Used mainly as a condiment, sesame seeds are actually made up of 50 percent heart-healthy monounsaturated fat. More important, the anti-oxidants in the seeds give them a significant impact in helping the body neutralize free radicals. In addition, sesame seeds have a high magnesium content to help steady nerves, and ½ cup of sesame seeds contains more than three times the calcium of a comparable measure of milk. Research suggests that sesamin, a compound found only in sesame seeds, can inhibit the production of arachidonic acid, the building block of the "bad" eicosanoids associated with heart disease, cancer, and arthritis.

Sesame seeds have a nutty, slightly sweet flavor and aroma that are enhanced by toasting. You can purchase them packaged in the spice section and in bulk quantity in Middle Eastern markets. Due to their high oil content, the seeds will quickly become rancid, so you should purchase them in small amounts and use them quickly. Seeds can be kept in an airtight container in a cool, dry place for up to three months, refrigerated for six months, or frozen for up to a year.

Did you know? We're all familiar with the phrase "Open sesame," the magic words used by Ali Baba to open the treasure cave in the classic tale *One Thousand and One Nights*. This word *sesame* may have been chosen as the code because sesame seeds were so common in Arab cuisine that anyone hearing the phrase would quickly forget it. Other interpretations suggest that the phrase was inspired by the way sesame seed pods burst open with a pop, much like the sound of a lock springing open.

Sesame Slaw with Arame

Serves 1

Block size

	Handful dried arame sea vegetable
2 Fat	2 teaspoons tahini
½ Carbohydrate	1 teaspoon umeboshi vinegar (Japanese plum vinegar)
	½ clove garlic, pressed
	Juice of ½ lemon
1 Fat	⅛ teaspoon olive oil
4 Protein	8 ounces extra-firm tofu, cubed
	1 tablespoon tamari or shoyu sauce
1 Fat	1 teaspoon sesame seeds
1 Carbohydrate	5 to 6 artichoke hearts, canned
1 Carbohydrate	¼ cup kidney beans
1 Carbohydrate	¼ cup black beans or chickpeas
½ Carbohydrate	Juice of ½ lemon
	Salt and pepper to taste
	Optional: 1 small sprig parsley, minced
	Optional: ⅛ teaspoon garlic salt
	12 leaves fresh lettuce

Cover arame in cold water, and soak overnight in refrigerator. (For fast preparation, simmer for 10 to 15
minutes in water.) Drain, refresh with cold water, drain
again. Chop arame coarsely. Combine tahini, vinegar,

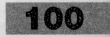

garlic, lemon juice, and olive oil and whisk with a fork. Add arame, toss until coated, and refrigerate, if desired, until ready to assemble dish. Toss tofu with tamari and sprinkle with sesame seeds. Set aside. Combine artichoke, beans, lemon juice, and seasonings in a bowl. Set aside. Place a thick bed of lettuce on a dinner plate. Place mound of arame in center. Encircle with tofu, artichoke, and bean mixture.

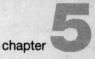

chapter 5

Eating Out or Dining In

Now that you've got the tools for making Zone meals and using the Top 100 foods, you may want some general pointers to help you stick with the Zone Diet in everyday life. Can you still go to restaurants and follow the Zone Diet? (The answer is a resounding yes!) What are some smart strategies for supermarket shopping? This chapter is a great resource guide for when you veer away a little from this book and start to improvise on your own.

I'm always drumming into your head that food is a drug, but I also want food to be the ultimate pleasure. You should be salivating over your Zone meals and treating yourself to a nice dinner at your favorite restaurant. The sheer enjoyment of food is an integral part of the Zone plan, and I don't want to deny you any of the eating pleasures you've experienced in the past. All you need to do is follow some simple guidelines, and you can eat the way you'd like and stay in the Zone. You *can* have it both ways!

DINING OUT: YOUR ZONE AWAY FROM HOME

Most restaurants simply provide too much food, especially low-quality carbohydrates like breads, pasta, and rice. It's cheaper for them to fill you up on starches, but it's hormonal disaster for you. Your goal is to transform your favorite restaurant meal into a Zone Meal. Follow these simple tips and it's automatic.

1. **Eat ahead of time.** Have a Zone snack less than two hours before you go to the restaurant. It's much easier to dine in the Zone and make the right food choices if your blood sugar is stable.

2. **Skip the bread.** When you are seated, simply ask your server not to bring any bread or rolls to the table. If you need something before your main course, have a glass of wine and a protein appetizer (like smoked salmon or shrimp cocktail). Sipping your wine, determine the protein entrée you plan to eat (such as grilled chicken or fish).

3. **Substitute for low-quality side dishes.** Ask your waiter if you can replace any side dishes that are low-quality carbohydrates (pasta, rice, grains, or other starches) with high-quality carbohydrates like steamed vegetables.

4. **Create a Zone-size meal.** When the meal arrives, cut a serving out of your protein entrée that's as big as the size and thickness of your palm. Ask your waiter to wrap the rest of your entrée up so you can take it home. Of course you still eat all of the high-quality carbohydrates that came with the entrée.

5. **Divvy up dessert**. If you want a rich dessert, eat only half and give the other half to your dining partner. Of course, if you opt for fresh fruit, you can eat the whole thing.

6. **Give yourself a little leeway**. Finally, if you consume too many carbohydrates or too many calories at a meal, don't worry that you've done irreparable damage. You can reset your hormonal system if you make sure your next meal is a Zone meal.

You can use these tips at any restaurant, but here are some additional hints for dining out in popular specialty restaurants.

Chinese
Forget the rice, and you have all the makings of a great Zone meal. Grilled fish or chicken, stir-fried chicken, or tofu dishes are great sources of protein. Choose a protein dish that's piled high with abundant levels of high-quality carbohydrates, such as vegetables, to accompany your high-protein choice.

Italian
This is always a potential Zone disaster because of the heaping amounts of pasta and bread piled on your plate. Try the chicken or fish entrées served with extra vegetables instead of pasta. Drizzle on some olive oil to enhance the flavor of your salads and cooked vegetables. If you want pasta, have it as a small side dish. I wouldn't recommend pasta, though, if you're planning on drinking wine, since you'll eat far too many carbohydrates to have a Zone meal.

Japanese
Japanese cuisine is more Zone balanced than what you typically find in a Chinese restaurant, but you still should avoid the rice. Fish and tofu entrées with abundant amounts of steamed vegetables are great. Even sushi is not a bad balance of protein and carbohydrate. (Helpful hint: A breaded protein dish like tempura is not a high-quality Zone protein choice.)

Mexican
This is another potential Zone disaster area because of the large amounts of low-quality carbohydrates, especially the chips, refried beans, rice, and tortillas. You can stay in the Zone, though, if you choose the chicken fajitas. Always ask for corn instead of flour tortillas to decrease your carbohydrate intake, and for extra vegetables in place of the rice or beans. Don't forget to dab on a little guacamole, which is a great source of monounsaturated fat.

French
If you're eating in a gourmet French restaurant, you'll probably be in Zone heaven. You'll be served a small serving of protein piled with plenty of crisp colorful vegetables lightly dressed in olive oil. Enjoy the wine and the meal.

Pizza Parlors
Yes, you *can* still eat pizza in the Zone. It's not the highest-quality meal you can find, but it's OK on occasion. Order the thin crust pizza instead of the thick crust and make sure you have a protein-rich topping like cheese, chicken or even anchovies. Then eat the topping of every slice, but only eat every other crust. To

make your pizza more satisfying, order extra vegetables as a topping.

Dining Out for Business Travelers

Eating on the road is one of the most stressful events for any business traveler, especially in new locales. At every meal use the basic guidelines outlined above. Here's a sample of some high-quality Zone meals that are always available regardless of where you're staying.

Breakfast
Egg-white omelette with a side order of oatmeal. This is the ultimate power breakfast. Just don't eat the toast and the hash brown potatoes.

Lunch
Chicken Caesar salad with fresh fruit for dessert.

Dinner
Grilled fish with extra vegetables in place of the starch. Have fresh fruit for dessert. Consider having a glass of wine with the dinner, and always pass on the rolls.

Road Snacks
Have 1 ounce of sliced turkey or low-fat cheese with half a piece of fruit.

Things to Avoid When Eating Out

Use common sense and avoid these low-quality Zone no-no's:

- Fatty meats (steaks, pork, lamb)
- Fried foods (including appetizers)

- French fries
- Chips
- Excessive amounts of starches (rice, pasta, and bread)
- Rich desserts (unless it is a very small portion size)

EATING IN: YOUR HOME ZONE

Surprisingly, most people only eat about 20 different food items. If you doubt me, just make a list. In fact, ask yourself how many of the Top 100 Zone Foods appear on that list. Chances are, you need to expand your culinary repertoire. Of course you can still eat your favorite protein, carbohydrate, and fat choices. Just add some new foods to the pot.

As you make your supermarket shopping list each week, make a point of including one or two new foods from my Top 100 list that you don't normally buy. Whether it's spinach to mix into your salad, asparagus to add to your omelette, or tofu to mix into your stir-fry vegetables, continually try new combinations. The recipes in this book are just suggestions. You can substitute different kinds of greens in your salads or steamed bok choy instead of broccoli. Whatever works for you.

YOUR GUIDE TO SUPERMARKET SHOPPING

Your supermarket shopping habits can make or break your commitment to the Zone. Stock your kitchen with the wrong kinds of foods, and you'll be left with no other choice but to eat them when the chips are down and you're famished. Your best bet? Leave the low-quality protein, carbohydrates, and fats where they should be: in someone else's kitchen.

Follow these steps to becoming a savvy supermarket shopper:

Step #1: Always go with a list. Go prepared with a list of high-quality Zone foods, and stick with that list. To help you stick with the list, make sure you don't shop when you're hungry. Eat a Zone meal or snack before you hit the supermarket.

Step #2: Stay mainly on the periphery. Ever notice that the fruits, vegetables, meat, fish, and dairy products are all found in the outer aisles? This is where you want to spend most of your time. Avoid the center aisles, which contain the processed foods like cereals, pasta, and snack foods. And of course, avoid the bakery at all costs.

Step #3: Make the produce section your foray into new adventures. OK, you may find it hard to pass up the new brand of chocolates that screams to you from its bright pink bag. But don't the bright red tomatoes also beckon? Or the deep purple blackberries? Go to a supermarket that displays appealing produce, free of bruises, mold, and brown spots. You'll be more tempted to dive into the colorful delights.

Step #4: Go for fresh meat and poultry rather than the deli counter. With the exception of cooked turkey breast, you can't find much high-quality protein at the deli. Head instead for the fish counter and the fresh meat choices. Just make sure that any beef or pork you buy is well trimmed, preferably a "select" grade that is low in saturated fat. You will probably still have to do some extra trimming of any separable fat to make it a good Zone protein choice. Realize that the deli turkey breast and chicken breast are of lower protein quality than fresh poultry.

Step #5: Consider buying organic produce. Organically grown fruits and vegetables are higher-quality Zone foods than nonorganically grown produce. This is because they are pesticide and herbicide free, and some research suggests that these chemicals can have negative effects on your hormonal systems. I realize that organically grown produce is more expensive, but I think the added cost is well worth the health benefit. Also consider buying your produce from a farm stand or one of the farmers' markets common in major cities. Although this produce isn't necessarily organically grown, it's fresher than the produce you find in the supermarket and thus probably has a higher nutrient content.

Frozen vs. Fresh

If you are like most people, you probably shop with the best intentions to buy fresh vegetables and fruits. Unfortunately, you've probably also come to realize that the shelf life of such fresh produce doesn't always conform to your daily schedule, and you may be sick of throwing away spoiled vegetables that you never got a chance to cook or fruit that has turned to mush. If this is the case, you have two options:

1. Consider purchasing fresh produce two to three times each week.

2. Use frozen fruits and vegetables.

The quality of frozen produce has dramatically increased over the years, and the shelf life will always be greater (usually about two months before freezer burn begins to set in). Furthermore frozen fruits and vegetables usually contain higher amounts of vitamins than fresh produce. This is because they are quick-frozen within hours after harvesting, while fresh produce may take many days after harvest to reach your local food distributor. From there you can expect a few more days before it gets to the supermarket and is bought and eaten by you. During this time the vitamin content of the food is constantly decreasing. By using frozen fruits and vegetables, you get maximum nutrition and convenience for the least cost.

Most people find it's easy to get stuck in a meal rut, preparing the same meals over and over again, week after week. It's easy, mindless, and less trouble than poring through new recipes. Still, I urge you to try a new food or two every week—or even every day if you can swing it. Just as you can make minor adjustments to your favorite meals to make them Zone-friendly, you can also make a few changes to your Zone meals to get the highest-quality foods. Within a few weeks, you'll have a formidable pharmacy of "drugs" to pick and choose from that will dramatically improve the quality of your life.

Zone Supplements

If you follow the Zone Diet and eat the Top 100 Zone Foods regularly, you can probably skip a multivitamin/mineral supplement since you'll be getting nearly all the nutrients you need through the foods you eat. (You can still pop a vitamin pill if you want to—as a form of cheap insurance—but you probably don't need it.)

I do, however, recommend that you supplement your diet daily with two vital nutrients that you probably don't get enough of—no matter how carefully you stick with the Zone Top 100. These are:

1. Fish oil (scientifically called long-chain Omega-3 fatty acids)

2. Vitamin E

WHY YOU NEED A FISH OIL SUPPLEMENT

Unless you eat one or two fish meals a day, you probably don't get enough long-chain Omega-3 fatty acids, which are found in fish oil. You need a sufficient amount of these fatty acids to keep your brain and cardiovascular and immune systems functioning at peak performance. Without understanding the full health benefits, your grandmothers and great-grandmothers had a sense of the importance of these fatty acids when they made their children take cod liver oil. Although high on the "yuck" factor for taste, cod liver oil is one of the best sources for long-chain Omega-3 fatty acids. The good news is that you no longer have to hold your nose and swallow to get enough Omega-3s. You can swallow a supplement in capsule form or eat a daily serving or two of a dark-fleshed fish like tuna, mackerel, or salmon.

I cannot emphasize enough how important it is for you to get long-chain Omega-3 fatty acids. The research is compelling. For instance, docosahexanenoic acid (DHA), a type of long-chain Omega-3 fatty acid, is found throughout the central nervous system and appears to play a primary role in how well your brain functions. A growing body of research has confirmed that infants who are deficient in DHA have deficient neurological responses and score lower on intelligence tests later in life. What's more, a substantial number of neurological conditions, such as depression, attention-deficit disorder, and schizophrenia, are linked to low levels of DHA in the bloodstream. More recently, researchers have found that patients with bipolar depression (the most difficult form of depression to treat) often respond dramatically to very high-dose supplementation with fish oils.

Yet another type of long-chain Omega-3 fatty acid is called eicosapentaenoic acid or EPA. This fatty acid has a powerful effect on decreasing inflammation and reducing the overproduction of "bad" eicosanoids. These "bad" eicosanoids are the true villains behind many chronic diseases such as heart disease, cancer, and arthritis, as well as a variety of neurological conditions such as multiple sclerosis, depression, and possibly Alzheimer's.

Taking fish oil supplements or eating dark-fleshed fish is a great way to up your intake of both of these long-chain Omega-3 fatty acids. However, this may not be an option if you're a vegetarian. Fortunately, biotechnology has provided a new option for vegetarians. Scientists have developed certain algae that produce a large amount of DHA-containing oils. Supplements using these DHA-rich oils solve the vegetarian's problem of getting enough DHA for optimal brain function. Your body can use DHA to make EPA, so you'll also get powerful anti-inflammatory benefits.

My Recommendation. Take 6 to 10 grams of fish oil per day, which supplies 2 to 3 grams of long-chain Omega-3 fatty acids. (Only about one-third of the fish oil in the capsule is actually composed of long-chain Omega-3 fatty acids.) Consuming up to 10 capsules per day may seem like a lot, but it's actually the same amount of Omega-3s contained in the tablespoon of cod liver oil that your grandmother doled out two generations ago. To ensure that the fish oil you consume is relatively free of toxins like PCBs, purchase a supplement that's cholesterol-free, since it's been more purified than regular-grade fish oil.

WHY YOU NEED VITAMIN E

No matter what diet you follow, chances are you're not consuming enough vitamin E to reap its full benefits. Seed oils are the richest source of vitamin E and are only consumed in moderation on the Zone Diet. Vitamin E is an anti-oxidant, which means that it neutralizes free radicals, which can destroy a healthy cell or induce inflammation. Vitamin E has been shown to have a dramatic effect on a variety of diseases ranging from heart disease to Alzheimer's. The scientific data is overwhelming for the increased intake of vitamin E in every diet.

Although the RDA for vitamin E is 10 IU for males and 8 IU for females, all the available clinical studies indicate that optimal health benefits from this vitamin only occur when vitamin E intake is greater than 100 IU per day.

My Recommendation. You should take a 400 IU daily supplement of vitamin E to ensure that you reap the maximum health benefits from this anti-oxidant.

DO YOU NEED OTHER SUPPLEMENTS?

As I mentioned earlier in the chapter, the answer is probably no—if you're using the Top 100 Zone Foods. If your carbohydrates consist mainly of grains and starches, however, you may indeed need to take more supplements. This is because low-quality carbohydrates, like pasta, bread, and rice, contain only scant amounts of vitamins and minerals. In a ranking of vitamins and minerals per gram of carbohydrate, vegetables would come out on top, with fruits coming in a strong second and grains a distant third. Just compare the nutrients found in specific foods from these categories in Table 6-1 (see page 314).

The Zone Food Science Ranking System reflects these differences in vitamins and minerals, giving broccoli an exceptionally high ranking on anti-oxidative capacity of 254, kiwi a good ranking of 51, and brown rice an extremely poor ranking of 0. As you can see, high-quality Zone foods are also great sources of vita-

Table 6-1

Comparison of Vitamin and Mineral Content in One Zone Block of Carbohydrate (9 Grams of Carbohydrates)

Carbohydrate	Amount	Vitamin A	Vitamin C	Folic Acid	Magnesium	Calcium	Fiber
Broccoli	3 cups	6,492	328	234.0	114	210.0	13.2
Kiwi	1	133	57	1.0	23	19.0	2.5
Rice, brown	⅓ cup	0	0	1.6	21	0.9	0.7

mins and minerals. The following list will give you a brief run-down of the health benefits of specific vitamins and minerals found in abundance in the Top 100 Zone Foods.

Vitamins

Vitamin A (Beta-Carotene)

Most of the vitamin A you get in food is in the form of beta-carotene, which your body breaks down into vitamin A. Beta-carotene is only one of hundreds of other carotenoids, which are powerful anti-oxidants. However, foods rich in beta-carotene are usually rich in a wide spectrum of other anti-oxidants. Some of the best sources of beta-carotene are fruits and vegetables that rank at the top of the Zone 100 list and include broccoli, spinach, kale, and berries.

Vitamins B_1, and B_2, and B_3

These water-soluble vitamins play a role in energy metabolism. One of the major misconceptions about the Zone Diet is that it doesn't provide enough B vitamins because it doesn't emphasize whole grains. While it's true that whole grains supply some B vitamins, you can also get plenty of vitamin B from high-quality Zone foods. For example, lean animal meat (especially pork) is very rich in vitamin B_1 (thiamin), and Zone Block for Zone Block it contains more B_1 than whole grains do. You can get plenty of B_2 and B_3 in meat, fish, poultry, and dairy products. Bottom line: If you are eating adequate amounts of high-quality Zone protein choices, you will be getting more than adequate levels of these B vitamins.

Vitamin B_6

This water-soluble B vitamin is found in soybeans, poultry, beef, pork, and fish (especially tuna and salmon). Although whole grains contain small amounts of B_6, more than 90 percent may be lost in the milling process. Unfortunately, more than 98 percent of the grain products consumed by Americans have been milled. Vitamin B_6 is critical for protein and essential fatty acid metabolism and for lowering elevated homocysteine levels, which can help prevent coronary artery disease.

Vitamin B_{12}

This vitamin, which is critical for neurological function and reduction of homocysteine levels, is only found in animal products. Fish and high-quality meat sources are good sources of this vitamin.

Vitamin C

This is the most well known of the water-soluble antioxidants. It is abundant in high-quality fruits and vegetables and virtually nonexistent in grains.

Vitamin D

This vitamin is essential to maintaining bone structure because it enhances absorption of calcium. You can get vitamin D from fatty fish such as salmon, sardines, and mackerel and vitamin D-fortified milk.

Folic Acid
This vitamin takes its name from the Latin word for "leaf" because it is found in green leafy vegetables. High-quality cruciferous vegetables are a great source of this vitamin, which helps reduce elevated homocysteine levels to prevent coronary artery disease.

Minerals

Calcium
Your best sources of calcium are dairy products and, to a lesser extent, high-quality vegetables such as broccoli, kale, spinach, and calcium-precipitated tofu. You need adequate levels of calcium to keep your bones strong and maintain a healthy nervous system.

Chromium
This mineral helps your body regulate insulin levels by reducing the amount of insulin needed to mop up excess blood sugar. High-quality meat, cheese, and legumes, such as soybeans, are all good sources of chromium.

Magnesium
Rich sources of magnesium include nuts and green vegetables, which are high-quality Zone foods. Magnesium plays a starring role in more than 300 enzymatic reactions and has recently been shown to have significant cardiovascular benefits.

Potassium
Avocado, broccoli, and citrus fruits are great sources of potassium. You need adequate levels of potassium in-

side your cells to maintain the electrical balance that is important for nerve conduction.

Selenium

Seafood, meat, and nuts contain the most abundant supplies of selenium. Vegetables and fruits contain less selenium and may contain varying amounts depending on soil conditions. Selenium is needed for the enzyme (glutathione peroxidase) that plays a key role in neutralizing free radicals.

Zinc

The best sources of zinc are high-quality protein products, including beef, chicken, and seafood. You need zinc to maintain a properly functioning immune system.

The next time you cringe over the price of fresh berries or organically grown apples, remember that they're providing a full dose of vitamins and minerals in the most natural way possible. (Not to mention their hidden trove of phytochemicals!) Given that Americans spend more than 13 billion dollars a year on dietary supplements, think how much we would save if all of us just ate more fruits and vegetables!

chapter **7**

Food and Hormones

Some 2,500 years ago, Hippocrates recognized the power of food when he said, "Let food be your medicine, and let medicine be your food." As we enter the twenty-first century, we can now update his wisdom by treating food as a powerful drug that can keep our hormones, especially insulin, within a magical Zone that keeps us healthy. To understand the science behind the Zone more fully, you first have to understand what hormones are and why insulin is the central character in this dietary drama.

INSULIN: YOUR JEKYLL AND HYDE HORMONE

Imagine hormones as biological messengers that transmit information almost instantaneously from one end of your body to the other. Since hormones must transmit messages to and from some 60 trillion cells, you can imagine how complex these interactions must be to maintain the flow of biological information. Among the hundreds of hormones discovered, insulin is probably the most widely studied because it is a hormone that tells your cells to store incoming nutrients necessary for your survival. Without an adequate supply of insulin, you would not be able to live. This is one reason why high-protein diets ultimately fail. You need to eat adequate amounts of carbohydrates in order to produce enough insulin for your cells to flourish.

You can have too much of a good thing, however, and this is the case with insulin. When you produce too much insulin (by eating too many carbohydrates or too many calories), you actually disrupt the flow of biological communication, and this can eventually cause your cells to go haywire. As a result, you put yourself at increased risk for developing a host of life-threatening diseases, such as heart disease, adult-onset (Type 2) diabetes, and cancer.

Because of its dual personality, I consider insulin to be the Jekyll and Hyde hormone. Just as the heroic Dr. Jekyll inadvertently turned himself into the evil Mr. Hyde, insulin can either sustain your life or destroy it. When maintained at adequate levels and kept under control, insulin acts like the selfless Dr. Jekyll, continuously delivering nutrients to cells in your body. When you eat too many carbohydrates, however, insulin's Dr. Jekyll persona quickly turns into Mr. Hyde—a raging hormonal monster that promotes fat storage, causing weight gain and a host of other health ills.

Excess insulin makes cellular communication difficult if not downright impossible. Like attempting a phone conversation with constant background noise over the wires, in the presence of excess insulin your cells get garbled hormonal messages. That causes them to start dividing too rapidly or begin producing too much or not enough of a particular substance. These cellular malfunctions that excess insulin causes can lead to many of the diseases associated with aging, such as obesity, heart disease, cancer, or adult-onset diabetes.

WHY THE ZONE WORKS

If you have excess levels of insulin, you need a drug to bring your levels back down to normal. But the drug of choice is a completely natural one: that's right, food. Yes, the very same substance that caused your insulin levels to soar in the first place can also help your levels return to normal. The Zone Diet is the antidote that will turn your insulin levels from Mr. Hyde back into Dr. Jekyll. Thus the hormonal key to a longer life lies in keeping insulin within the Zone: not too high, nor too low.

About 25 percent of the U.S. population are genetically lucky individuals who are able to eat lots of low-quality carbohydrates and never produce too much insulin. The other 75 percent of us are genetically predisposed to developing insulin resistance. This happens when your muscle cells don't respond well to insulin's signal to store blood sugar. When this happens, your body continues to pump out more and more insulin in an effort to get your muscle cells to pay attention to insulin's message. Eventually, in the face of this continual bombardment of insulin, the receptors for insulin on your muscle cells become increasingly dysfunctional, forcing your body to make even more insulin to try to get its message (store blood sugar) heard. Meanwhile your fat cells hear insulin's message loud and clear, and they continue to store fat very effectively. Over time your insulin levels become constantly elevated, a condition called hyperinsulinemia. Once you develop hyperinsulinemia, cellular communication throughout your body becomes garbled, and this marks the beginning of many chronic disease conditions.

How can you tell if you are genetically predisposed to make excess insulin? Take this very simple test: Eat a big pasta meal at lunch, and then see how you feel three hours later. If you can barely keep your eyes open, then you are a genetically ticking time bomb. The good news is that the amount and type of food you eat can control your genetic predisposition toward insulin resistance.

Keep in mind that chronically elevated insulin levels (hyperinsulinemia) precede the development of obesity, Type 2 diabetes, and heart disease. If you suspect that your dietary habits have wreaked havoc on your insulin levels, you can have a simple blood test to see whether your insulin levels are elevated.

Your doctor should order a fasting insulin blood test. To be in the Zone, your insulin levels should be between 5 and 10 uU/ml. If your levels are higher than 15 uU/ml, you have hyperinsulinemia, which means you're at greatly increased risk of developing obesity, Type 2 diabetes, cardiovascular disease, and cancer.

Fortunately, you have a proven treatment that can reduce elevated insulin levels within a few weeks: the Zone Diet. Use the Top 100 Zone Foods on the Zone Diet, and you can begin to reverse hyperinsulinemia and insulin resistance within a few days.

GLUCAGON: YOUR ANTI-INSULIN HORMONE

In addition to controlling your insulin levels, the Zone Diet can help you control another hormone called glucagon, which has the opposite effect of insulin. Just as carbohydrates trigger the release of insulin, protein stimulates the release of glucagon. Whereas insulin tells your cells to take sugar out of the bloodstream and store it, glucagon tells your liver to release stored sugar for the brain. Your body strives to maintain a balance of insulin and glucagon so that the brain gets all the fuel it needs without an overproduction of insulin, which can give rise to obesity and chronic disease.

If you've ever experienced the lightheadedness and shakiness caused by hypoglycemia (low blood sugar), you know how much your brain relies on adequate levels of blood sugar to function. When you're hypoglycemic, your brain virtually commands you to eat any carbohydrate in sight to increase blood sugar levels. Many people call these carbohydrate cravings, and you may have experienced them yourself. They occur, not because you are a weak-willed person, but because you made the wrong hormonal choice at your last meal.

What you may not realize is that the more carbohydrates you eat, the more likely you are to become hypoglycemic. Too many carbohydrates can cause excessive amounts of insulin to be released, which drives down blood sugar. As a result, your blood sugar levels dip far below what they were before you had your meal. This makes you tired and leads you on a search for quick energy in the form of more carbohydrates, which sets you on a vicious cycle.

Contrary to what you might think, the best way to get a handle on hypoglycemia is not to feed it with sugar. You need to prevent it from occurring in the first place by maintaining a balance of protein to carbohydrate at each meal. This is because protein stimulates the release of glucagon, which maintains blood sugar levels for the brain. What's more, glucagon acts like a hormonal brake that inhibits excess insulin secretion. By maintaining relatively constant levels of glucagon, you will control insulin levels with far greater ease.

Thus you will help your body achieve the balance it seeks between insulin and glucagon.

By spreading your protein intake throughout the day on the Zone Diet, you will constantly produce glucagon to stabilize your insulin levels. At the same time, you should never eat too much protein at one meal. This is important because your body will convert any excess protein to fat. That's why I recommend eating no more than 3 or 4 ounces of low-fat protein at any given meal.

You should now be able to see why eating a balanced ratio of protein to carbohydrate at every meal and snack makes good hormonal sense and will give you a healthy level of both insulin and glucagon in your bloodstream for the next four to six hours.

EICOSANOIDS: YOUR MASTER HORMONES

Eicosanoids are the last group of diet-induced hormones that play a role in reaching the Zone. They are extremely short-lived and difficult to study. Nonetheless, the 1982 Nobel Prize in Medicine was awarded for understanding the critical role that eicosanoids play in chronic disease. Although you may never have heard of them, these hormones play a huge role in determining whether you'll be healthy or stricken with chronic illnesses like heart disease, cancer, and diabetes.

Like insulin, eicosanoids are two-faced and can be either "good" or "bad" depending on their structure. Eating too many low-quality fats rich in Omega-6 fatty acids (like soybean and corn oil) can trigger the overproduction of "bad" eicosanoids. Increased insulin also increases the production of "bad" eicosanoids.

You can reduce the production of "bad" eicosanoids and pump up the production of "good" eicosanoids by eating high-quality fats rich in long-chain Omega-3 fatty acids (such as fish or fish oil supplements) and by stabilizing your insulin levels on the Zone Diet. Control your eicosanoids, and you essentially become the master over the inner workings of your body. This is pretty heady stuff; you can read more about these hormones in *The Zone* and *The Anti-Aging Zone*.

To *control these three hormonal systems (insulin, glucagon, and eicosanoids) you need dietary balance and moderation, which are the hallmarks of the Zone Diet.*

THE HORMONAL BENEFITS OF REDUCING CALORIES

As you embark on this hormonal balancing act, you need to remember one thing: It's not just the balance of foods you eat, it's also the amount. You can eat the perfect ratio of carbohydrates to protein to fat, but if you eat too much food in general, you are not going to stay in the Zone. This is because the amount of calories you eat also plays a key role in determining your insulin levels. Eating too many calories at a meal triggers the release of excess insulin. For this reason, the Zone Diet is designed to enable you to consume the fewest calories possible without feeling hungry or deprived, because your brain is getting a constant and stable supply of blood sugar. Using the Top 100 Zone Foods and following the Zone Diet enables you to maintain excellent mental and physical performance with maximum nutrition all with the least number of calories. At *every* meal, you should plan to eat just enough protein (the amount you can fit on the palm of your hand) to maintain your strength and your immune system and just the right amount of carbohydrates (two to three servings of vegetables and fruits) to stabilize your insulin levels. And don't forget to add a dash of heart-healthy monounsaturated fat.

By following that simple dietary advice, you will be getting the right amount of calories—not too many and not too few. Sixty years of scientific research have shown that such calorie restriction is the only proven way to reverse the aging process. But rather than using the term calorie *restriction,* I prefer to call it calorie *conversion.* You conserve the number of calories you consume at every meal by eating the highest-quality Zone foods. This will give you the maximum number of vitamins, minerals, and other micronutrients in the fewest calories. It's no wonder, then, that you'll live longer and better using the Top 100 Zone Foods and following the Zone Diet.

Eating an abundance of fruits and vegetables on the Zone Diet (and relatively little grains), you have to put forth a lot of effort to consume too many calories in the form of carbohydrates. This is because, ounce for ounce, vegetables contain much fewer carbohydrates per serving than starches, pasta, bread, or grains. For instance, 1 cup of pasta contains as many carbohydrates as 12 cups of steamed broccoli. You know how easy it is to eat a cup of pasta, but have you ever attempted to eat 12 cups of broccoli? Since it's so easy to overconsume pasta and other high-density carbohydrates, I treat them as condiments on the Zone Diet. Table 7-1, on page 326, shows you a comparison between high-density and low-density carbohydrates. Each of these foods contains about 10 grams of carbohydrates—yet they have very different serving sizes.

You can see that by eating primarily fruits and vegetables, you'll have a much easier time keeping your in-

Table 7-1.
Volume Comparison of Different Carbohydrates Providing
One Zone Food Block (9 Grams of Carbohydrate)

Source	One Zone Block
A. Low-Density Carbohydrates	
Broccoli	3 cups
Peppers	2 cups
Zucchini	2 cups
String beans	1½ cups
B. Intermediate-Density Carbohydrates	
Strawberries	1 cup
Peaches	1 cup
Oranges	½ fruit
Apples	½ fruit
C. High-Density Carbohydrates	
Bread	½ slice
Cereal	¼ cup
Pasta	¼ cup
Rice	⅓ cup

sulin levels under control when you combine these carbohydrates with the right amount of protein. You'll also be treating yourself to a healthy dose of anti-oxidants, since fruits and vegetables pack far more of these nutrients than grains. These superhealthy carbohydrates are the secret behind controlling your raging hormones. Once you've got a handle on the hormones, you've got the wonder drug you need to live a longer and healthier life. And then the Zone will have fulfilled its promise.

chapter 8

The Zone vs. Other Diets

OK admit it. You've tried other diets. Maybe you embraced no-fat, high-carbohydrate diets in the '80s and turned to high-protein diets in the '90s. Perhaps you spent two weeks eating nothing but grapefruit, or you consumed so many bowls of cabbage soup that you'll never look at another cabbage again. Chances are, you found that your weight-loss success was followed by dismal failure as you regained the lost weight and then some. All I can say is you're not alone.

As Americans continue their search for a quick-fix way to lose weight, they continue to grow fatter with each passing year. More than half of us are overweight, and one-third of us are downright obese. I can't say I'm surprised that none of these fad weight-loss diets work to help you lose weight over the long haul. The reason is simple: both high-carbohydrate and high-protein diets will eventually give rise to excess insulin production. Remember that it's excess insulin that makes you fat and keeps you fat.

These unbalanced eating plans upset the balance of

insulin (your glucose storage hormone) and glucagon (your glucose mobilization hormone). Diets composed primarily of high-density, low-quality carbohydrates like bread and pasta cause an immediate surge in insulin levels. Diets high in protein with very low amounts of carbohydrates put your body into an unnatural state called ketosis, which can eventually cause fat cells to adapt to become "fat magnets" that retain any incoming fat, causing you to gain excess weight over time.

But these are both fad diets, so you probably expect them to have a catch. You may be surprised to hear, however, that even the dietary recommendations made by the U.S. Department of Agriculture (USDA) can cause you to gain weight if you are genetically predisposed to make lots of insulin (as 75 percent of Americans are). The USDA's Food Pyramid tells you that high-density carbohydrates in the form of bread, cereal, rice, and pasta should be the centerpiece of your diet. Yet these are the very foods that trigger excess insulin production, which makes you fat and keeps you fat. By now you should realize that the politically correct carbohydrates, which you have been told are great for your health, are actually some of the most hormonally incorrect foods you can eat.

THE USDA FOOD PYRAMID VS. THE ZONE FOOD PYRAMID

Once you understand the role of insulin in obesity and then study closely the recommendations made in the USDA Food Pyramid, you'll be astounded that our government would continue to recommend this type of diet. If you follow the USDA recommendations, you'll be virtually guaranteeing an increase in your insulin levels and quite possibly an increase in your body fat! Consider this: The government recommends eating 6 to 11 servings each day of high-density, low-quality carbohydrates like pasta, mashed potatoes, and bagels. Using the serving sizes recommended by the USDA, this amounts to approximately 220 grams of carbohydrates each day. The government also recommends eating a minimum of 3 to 5 small servings of fruits and vegetables each day. This would give you an additional 35 grams of carbohydrates (based on 2 servings of fruit and 3 servings of vegetables). Thus you would get a whopping 255 grams of carbohydrates each day—more than what you'd get in 1¼ cups of table sugar or six candy bars.

Now let's compare this with the Zone Diet. On the Zone, you get 10 to 15 daily servings of high-quality fruits and vegetables (three times the amount recommended by the USDA). Even with these extra servings of fruits and vegetables, you still get only about 110 grams of carbohydrates a day. In addition, you'll probably have 2 servings a day of a high-density carbohydrate, which would give you another 20 grams of carbohydrate, providing a grand total of 130 grams of carbohydrate. Thus on the Zone Diet you consume about half the amount of carbohydrates you'd get on the USDA diet, but you get to eat three times as many high-quality carbohydrates. That makes the Zone a pretty great nutritional bargain!

Reducing your carbohydrate consumption by almost half on the Zone Diet will give you a similar reduction in insulin secretion. Take a look at the illustrated USDA Food Pyramid and Zone Food Pyramid (see page 331). You'll quickly see the differences in terms of which foods are emphasized (the ones at the base of each pyramid). You'll see how the USDA Food Pyramid is virtually guaranteed to increase insulin lev-

Table 8-1
Comparison of Total Carbohydrate Consumption Following
the USDA Food Pyramid or the Zone Diet

	Servings	Carbohydrate (grams)
A. USDA Recommendations		
Grains	11	220
Fruits	2	20
Vegetables	3	15
Total	16	255
B. Zone Recommendations		
Grains	2	40
Fruits	5	50
Vegetables	10	50
Total	17	140

els, which will make you fatter, more likely to develop heart disease, and more likely to die a premature death.

THE FAILURE OF HIGH-CARBOHYDRATE DIETS

As I've said again and again, the more carbohydrates you eat, the more insulin you produce. Yet some nutritionists call for even more carbohydrates in our diets as an answer to the obesity epidemic. Low-quality carbohydrates like pasta, bread, bagels, rice, and other starches are very dense in carbohydrates, and eating more of these foods will increase the levels of insulin in your body. That's why these carbohydrates fall very low on my list when they are put through my Zone Food Quality Ranking System. You're probably puzzled

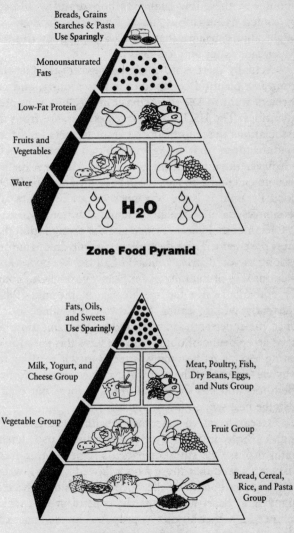

Zone Food Pyramid

Breads, Grains
Starches & Pasta
Use Sparingly

Monounsaturated
Fats

Low-Fat Protein

Fruits and
Vegetables

Water

H_2O

USDA Food Pyramid

Fats, Oils,
and Sweets
Use Sparingly

Milk, Yogurt, and
Cheese Group

Meat, Poultry, Fish,
Dry Beans, Eggs,
and Nuts Group

Vegetable Group

Fruit Group

Bread, Cereal,
Rice, and Pasta
Group

about why these low-quality carbohydrates would still be touted as nutritious foods. I am, too. In fact, you might almost believe that there's a conspiracy to make Americans fatter and less healthy.

Actually there is no conspiracy except the fact that grain is a plentiful commodity in this country, and our farmers want to keep growing it and selling it in huge quantities. The USDA often receives pressure from the associations that represent the grain farmers (and food manufacturers that make grain-based food products) whenever the government comes out with new dietary recommendations. In fact, it can be argued that the USDA Food Pyramid is based too much on grain politics and economics and not enough on sound nutritional science.

High-carbohydrate diets make the presumption that fat is the enemy. These diets allow carbohydrate gluttony as long as you deprive yourself of all fat. We now know that this way of thinking is completely wrong. Our country embarked on a fat-free lifestyle in the mid-1980s. Currently we are eating the lowest percentage of fat since the nineteenth century, and at the same time we have an epidemic of obesity. So we have this paradox of eating less fat yet becoming fatter. Somewhere along the way we forgot that the best way to fatten cattle is to feed them lots and lots of low-fat grain. It turns out that is also the best way to fatten humans.

Research on the assumed health benefits of the high-carbohydrate, very low-fat diets also hasn't panned out. One study of patients with existing heart disease showed that those who followed a very low-fat, very high-carbohydrate diet for five years had twice as many fatal heart attacks as the control group, which followed a higher-fat diet as proposed by the American Heart Association. This led the Nutrition Committee of the American Heart Association to conclude:

Because very low-fat diets represent a radical departure from current prudent dietary guidelines, such diets must be proven both advantageous and safe before national recommendations can be issued.

At the very least, you should avoid these types of very low-fat, very high-carbohydrate diets until there is any confirmatory evidence to suggest that such a radical diet will not increase fatal heart attacks when compared with higher-fat diets.

THE MYTH OF THE HIGH-PROTEIN DIET

In the face of the unmitigated disaster that high-carbohydrate diets have brought to our waistlines, millions of Americans have desperately turned to high-protein diets. Although these diets have been around for more than 30 years, they made a comeback in the mid-1990s as fat-free eating fell out of favor.

First of all, let me say once again that the Zone is not a high-protein diet. Yes, it includes more protein (but not excessive amounts) than the high-carbohydrate diets that many Americans are on, but it also gives you a balance of other macronutrients like carbohydrates and fats. Furthermore, since you are eating more carbohydrates than protein on the Zone Diet, it is very hard to call it a high-protein diet.

High-protein diets, on the other hand, contain very few carbohydrates and consist predominantly of protein and fat. There is no limit on the amount of protein you can eat, and there is no distinction made between artery-clogging saturated fat and heart-healthy monounsaturated fat and eicosanoid-friendly Omega-3 fatty acids. Basically, these high-protein diets make no distinction between a fatty T-bone steak and a grilled salmon steak. The advocates of high-protein diets ask you to abandon dietary common sense to eat all the fatty protein you want. But you should never have to give up good nutrition—no matter how hefty the promise of weight loss.

In fact, many people will ultimately *gain* weight on high-protein diets. Yes, it is true that millions of people have initially lost weight on these diets over the past 30 years, but the same millions have all gained the weight back and more. Although you may lose weight rapidly (much of it water) during the first few weeks, you may find yourself putting on pounds after three to six months on this type of diet. This is because of the metabolic adaptations your body is trying to make to this abnormal type of diet.

Quite frankly, you can't chow down on all the protein you please without expecting any negative health ramifications. Whenever you fail to eat adequate amounts of carbohydrates, your body goes into a state of ketosis in which it makes high levels of ketone bodies. Ketone bodies are the by-product of the incomplete metabolism of fats, which requires a certain level of carbohydrates in the liver. (Many critics of the Zone have charged that the Zone Diet puts you into ketosis. That's impossible because you always eat more carbohydrates than protein, making it impossible to generate ketones.)

Ketosis is simply not a balanced or natural state for your body to be in. As a result, your fat cells begin to adapt to become "fat magnets" over time. This actually causes you to gain weight rapidly three to six months into these types of diets. As if this weren't bad enough, eating gobs of saturated fat on a high-protein diet indirectly alters the insulin receptors on your muscle cells, making them less responsive to insulin. As a result, you wind up with increased insulin levels—the primary reason that you became fat in the first place.

It's no wonder so many people find themselves gaining weight after taking a turn around the high-protein-diet dance floor. Not to mention the fact that they also increase the risk for heart disease, since continued ketosis can have a damaging effect on your arteries. History will continue to repeat itself as more and more people initially lose weight on these high-protein diets and then gain the weight right back again.

THE AMERICAN HEART ASSOCIATION DIET

This diet restricts cholesterol and saturated fat intake, but like the USDA Food Pyramid, it relies too heavily on high-density carbohydrates like grains, starches, and pasta. As a result of increased carbohydrate intake, your insulin levels can increase. Ironically, the number-one risk factor that predicts future heart disease is increased insulin levels. Thus this diet can actually increase your risk of heart disease and diabetes by increasing your insulin levels if you are among the 75 percent who are genetically predisposed to insulin resistance.

THE MEDITERRANEAN DIET

This diet was used in the Lyon Diet Heart Study, which demonstrated a dramatic reduction in the number of fatal heart attacks. In this study, patients who had already had one heart attack followed either the Mediterranean diet or the American Heart Association diet for four years. Those who followed the Mediterranean diet experienced a 65 percent reduction in fatal heart attacks compared with those who followed the American Heart

Association diet. Like the Zone Diet, the Mediterranean diet gives you 30 percent of your calories from heart-healthy monounsaturated fat and Omega-3 fatty acids. It also stresses the increased consumption of fruits and vegetables and low-fat protein like fish, just like the Zone.

The Mediterranean diet, however, still pushes too many high-density grains and starches like pasta (which increase insulin levels) and doesn't include nearly as many fruit and vegetable servings as the Zone. You simply can't achieve the same degree of insulin control on the Mediterranean diet as you can following the Zone Diet. For that reason, I consider the Mediterranean diet to be a poor dietary cousin to the Zone.

Following the Zone, you consume more anti-oxidants and you have superior insulin control compared with any other diet. This translates into greater fat loss and greater longevity. Considering all the health benefits of the Zone, why would anyone want to try any other dietary program?

chapter 9

Motivation for a Lifetime in the Zone

Any diet you follow is only as good as the benefits you derive from it. Sure, we'd all like to eat anything at any time in any portion that we please. But this will shorten our lifespan, make us more prone to chronic disease, and cause us to plump up to look like the Pillsbury Dough Boy. Obviously, these consequences aren't what we want to achieve.

To embark on a dietary change that you can stick with for the rest of your life requires a significant motivational push. For many of us, that push comes from fear, because it is fear that usually prompts a call to action. For most baby boomers, that fear is called aging. I myself made the switch to the Zone Diet because I had a fear of dying prematurely from a heart attack.

The concept of the Zone goes directly to the core of reversing aging: improved hormonal control. When you think about which benefits of the Zone will be most meaningful to you, begin to list the greatest fears you have about aging.

Many people would say that their greatest fear is

for their brain to fail before their body does. Many also fear that their skin will look older than their true age. The Zone can help allay these fears by keeping you thinking and looking young. Let me tell you how.

The best way to keep your brain young is to keep it continually supplied with two things it needs to function well: oxygen and blood sugar. Without either, your brain will soon resemble a prune, as your nerve cells languish and die without these nutrients. To keep a stable supply of blood sugar, you have to be continually in the Zone. If you add a healthy dose of fish oil, to provide long-chain Omega-3 fatty acids, and simultaneously reduce the amount of Omega-6 fatty acids (from vegetable oils), you'll increase the flow of oxygen to the brain by making more "good" eicosanoids. Do both of these by following the Zone using high-quality foods and supplementing your diet with extra fish oil, and you will increase mental acuity and keep your brain humming along in a youthful state.

Your skin is no different from your brain, as it, too, needs constant hormonal attention. In particular, you need to increase blood flow and decrease inflammation (by increasing long-chain Omega-3 fatty acids and decreasing Omega-6 fatty acids) to keep your skin supple and wrinkle-free. The increased blood flow to your skin from following the Zone Diet will give it a rosy, healthy-looking glow. This increased blood flow to the skin also promotes the increased synthesis of collagen and elastin in your skin, which keeps it supple and smooth. Finally, by decreasing inflammation in the skin, you reduce the number-one cause of wrinkle formation: the microscarring of collagen fibers.

Reducing inflammation is one of the key factors for a better life. The two best ways are to consume high-quality Zone carbohydrates (rich in anti-oxidants) and to decrease the production of "bad" eicosanoids. This is why I minimize the amount of Omega-6 fatty acids in the Zone Diet. They are the building blocks of those "bad" eicosanoids that decrease blood flow (to either the brain or the skin) and promote inflammation. This is why you need to pay close attention to the quality rating of the fat you choose on the Zone Diet.

You already know that by lowering excess insulin levels the Zone Diet can decrease your risk of being overweight or having a chronic disease condition like heart disease or diabetes. I have talked about these benefits throughout the book. But you are probably even more concerned with how old you're going to look in the mirror each morning and how easily you'll retain your long-term and short-term memory. Regardless of how you prioritize your health concerns, know that getting sick, gaining weight, losing mental clarity, and looking wrinkled do not have to be inevitable results of the aging process.

You *can* grow old gracefully if you stay in the Zone. You don't need to turn to medications to control heart disease or diabetes if you have the appropriate eating habits. Nor will you need a facelift or liposuction. We'd all love to take a pill or have a medical procedure rather than revamp our habits. Unfortunately, these remedies only address the symptoms, not the real cause of aging, and they always have side effects. In addition, they can never offer the wide range of health benefits you'll find in the Zone.

Besides addressing your greatest fears about aging, the Zone Diet will give you some immediate pay-offs. If you are willing to follow the Zone for only a week, you will observe three immediate benefits:

1. Better thinking
2. Better performance
3. Better looks

The same hormonal control that gives you long-term health benefits also gives you these immediate benefits day in and day out. By stabilizing your blood sugar levels throughout the day, you will find that your mental functioning will rapidly improve. By lowering your insulin levels, you'll be able to tap into excess body fat to burn for an unlimited source of energy. Now you can come home from work and have enough energy to take a refreshing bike ride or play tag with your kids where you once used to just plop into a chair in front of the TV.

Even more good news: the weight loss you achieve is virtually all fat, so you'll find your clothes fitting better and your body looking more fit and toned.

The key to living a better life comes from controlling your hormones through the foods you eat. You have, in your hands, the Top 100 Zone Foods for the Zone Diet. Although the Zone will continue to evolve as new research comes to light, you pretty much know what it takes to achieve good health. Get a balance of protein, carbohydrates, and fat, and eat all foods in moderation. Above all, choose the highest-quality foods you can find—those that naturally contain the most disease-fighting nutrients. Do this, and you've got the ideal "drug" for the twenty-first century. Use this drug wisely, and you will live long and prosper.

Appendix A

Technical Support

I hope you now realize that the Zone Diet may be your most powerful tool for improving daily performance (both mental and physical), losing excess body fat, and living a longer and healthier life. Although I use the name Zone Diet, this is not a short-term program so much as a lifelong food management system for better health through enhanced hormonal control using the foods you already enjoy eating.

This is the eighth book I have written about my Zone technology. My first book, *The Zone*, was written primarily for cardiovascular physicians to educate them about the power that food has to alter hormone levels—specifically, how insulin, glucagon, and eicosanoid hormones vary depending on how much protein, fat, and carbohydrates you eat. *The Zone*, however, is not the best introduction for a beginner. To understand how simple the Zone technology is to follow, I strongly recommend reading the recently published *A Week in the Zone*. *Zone Perfect Meals in Minutes* and *Mastering the Zone* then provide more details about how to use the Zone Diet.

Once you understand basic Zone logic, you can refer back to *The Zone* to better understand the biochemistry behind it. If you really want to learn how to reverse aging and extend your lifespan, I strongly recommend reading *The Anti-Aging Zone*. This is my manifesto of the entire Zone technology I've developed. Although *The Anti-Aging Zone* is more complex than *The Zone,* it provides the information and motivation to make the Zone Diet your lifelong ally to increase and enhance your longevity by reversing the aging process.

Although each of my books represents the latest research on the complex relationship between diet and hormonal response, the field is constantly changing. You can keep abreast of the changing Zone technology by accessing my web site: *www.drsears.com,* which reviews the latest research on this rapidly evolving field. I am constantly updating this site with new recipes (many of them vegetarian), new research information, and simple tips to make the Zone Diet incredibly easy to follow on a lifelong basis.

The mission of my web site is to serve as a clearinghouse for information not only about the Zone Diet but also about the latest hormonal research, how diet can affect various hormones, and the impact of those hormones on your longevity. Since this information is rapidly changing, *drsears.com* should be your primary Internet destination to help you digest (no pun intended) the latest nutritional news. You can also email me via my web site with comments and suggestions about the Zone program. If you would like to receive a free Zone Reference Guide filled with useful information showing you how simple and easy Zone living can be, please call my toll-free number, 1–800–404–8171.

All About Carbohydrates

Since the Zone Diet is about insulin control, you have to realize that not all carbohydrates affect insulin equally. Every complex carbohydrate must be broken down into simple sugars and will eventually enter the bloodstream as glucose, which in turn will have a stimulatory effect on insulin secretion. Fiber (both soluble and insoluble) cannot be broken down into simple sugars, and therefore it will have no impact on insulin. Taking this into account, I developed the concept of a food's insulin-stimulating carbohydrate content. Simply stated, this is the total amount of carbohydrate a food source contains minus its fiber content (which is usually included in determining the total amount of carbohydrates).

If a carbohydrate source (such as pasta) has very little fiber content, then virtually all of its listed carbohydrate content will be insulin-stimulating carbohydrate. On the other hand, if a carbohydrate source is rich in fiber (such as broccoli), then its insulin-stimulating carbohydrate content will be significantly reduced. This means that more volume of a fiber-rich carbohydrate source must be consumed to have the same impact on insulin secretion as a much smaller volume of a fiber-poor carbohydrate (see Table B-1 below).

Table B-1
Amounts of Insulin-Stimulating Carbohydrates in Various Foods by Volume

Food	Volume	Total Carbs (g)	Fiber (g)	Insulin-Stimulating Carbs (g)
Pasta	1 cup	40	2	38
Apple	1 medium	20	4	16
Broccoli	1 cup	7	4	3

You can quickly see that you would have to eat a tremendous volume of broccoli (approximately 12 cups) to have the same impact on insulin as eating a relatively small amount of cooked pasta. This is why starches and grains are considered high-density carbohydrates, whereas fruits are medium-density carbohydrates and vegetables are low-density carbohydrates. The Zone Diet relies heavily on low-density carbohydrates, so large volumes of food must be consumed in order to have an appreciable impact on insulin. This is also why high-density carbohydrates are used in moderation on the Zone Diet, because very small volumes can stimulate excess insulin production.

ZONE BLOCKS OF CARBOHYDRATE

Zone Food Blocks are simply a way of putting various carbohydrates on an equal footing in terms of their insulin-

stimulating effect. I define a Zone Block of carbohydrate as
a volume containing 9 grams of insulin-stimulating carbohydrate. So let's return to the above example and determine the approximate amount of Zone Carbohydrate
Food Blocks in each of the sources (see Table B-2 below).

Table B-2
Zone Food Block Calculations

Food	Volume	Insulin-Stimulating Carbs (g)	Approx. Zone Carb Blocks
Pasta	1 cup	38	38/9 = 4
Apple	1 medium	16	16/9 = 2
Broccoli	1 cup	3	3/9 = ⅓

These numbers aren't too easy to remember, so I simplified them by normalizing the volume of the carbohydrate
source required to make one Zone Carbohydrate Food
Block. This is accomplished by dividing the volume of the
carbohydrate source in Table B-2 by the number of Zone
Carbohydrate Food Blocks in that same source. Then you
round that number to an approximate volume that you can
easily remember, as shown in Table B-3, below.

Table B-3
Zone Carbohydrate Block Calculations Simplified

Food	Zone Blocks in a Volume	Volume for One Zone Block
Pasta	1 cup has 4 Zone Blocks	¼ cup
Apple	1 medium has 2 Zone Blocks	½ apple
Broccoli	1 cup has ⅓ Zone Block	3 cups

Now you have a way to compare carbohydrates directly according to their ability to stimulate insulin secretion. A more complete listing of Zone Food Blocks containing carbohydrates is found in Appendix C.

THE CONCEPTS OF GLYCEMIC INDEX AND GLYCEMIC LOAD

One of the major nutrition breakthroughs was the development of the concept of the glycemic index. Previously it was thought that there were only simple and complex carbohydrates. The simple ones would enter the bloodstream rapidly, whereas the complex carbohydrates would be slowly broken down, thus providing sustained release over time. From this seemingly reasonable concept came the "nutritional wisdom" that eventually led to the development of the USDA Food Pyramid.

But when researchers began to ask whether such simplistic thinking was justified, they found that lo and behold, it wasn't. Some simple carbohydrates, such as fructose, entered the bloodstream as glucose very slowly. On the other hand, some complex carbohydrates, such as potatoes, entered the bloodstream at a faster rate than table sugar. The explanation of this apparent paradox led to the concept of the glycemic index.

The glycemic index is a measure of the entry rates of various carbohydrate sources into the bloodstream. The faster their rate of entry, the greater the effect on insulin secretion. There are three factors that affect the glycemic index of a particular carbohydrate. The first is the amount of fiber (and especially soluble fiber) a carbohydrate contains; the second is the amount of fat it contains (the more fat consumed with the carbohydrate, the slower the rate of entry into the bloodstream); the third is the composition of the complex carbohydrate itself: the greater the amount of glucose it contains, the higher the glycemic index; the more fructose it contains, the lower the glycemic index. This is because fructose cannot enter the bloodstream without first being converted into glucose. This is a relatively slow process that takes place in the liver.

With time the glycemic index became the new fashionable guideline to determine which carbohydrates to eat. However, the glycemic index had significant experimental problems in dealing with low-density carbohydrates, such as vegetables.

The difficulties arose because determination of the glycemic index requires that a sufficient amount of carbohydrate (usually 50 grams) be consumed. But it is simply too difficult to consume this amount of carbohydrate from most vegetables at a sitting. For instance this would require consuming about 16 cups of steamed broccoli. As a result, nearly all the glycemic index work has been done with grains, starches, and some fruits, and virtually nothing is known about the glycemic index of the low-density vegetables that are the backbone of the Zone Diet.

These difficulties have given rise to a more sophisticated concept known as the glycemic load, which is far more important than the glycemic index in determining the insulin output of a meal. The glycemic load is the actual amount of insulin-stimulating carbohydrates consumed multiplied by its glycemic index. This reflects the reality that a small volume of high-glycemic carbohydrates has the same impact on insulin as a large volume of low-glycemic carbohydrates. Therefore, eating too many low-glycemic carbohydrates can still have a major effect on increased insulin production. For example, black beans have a low glycemic index because of their high fiber content. However, they are also very dense in carbohydrate content. As a result, eating too many black beans at a meal can have a great stimulatory effect on insulin.

Ultimately, a healthy diet is obtained through insulin moderation, which can best be achieved by primarily consuming low-density carbohydrates that also have a low glycemic index. That means eating a lot of vegetables. To illustrate this concept, Table B-4, below, examines three distinct carbohydrate sources in the volumes in which they are typically consumed. The glycemic load is the product of the number of grams of insulin-stimulating carbohydrate times the glycemic index for that carbohydrate. The lower the glycemic load number, the lower the insulin stimulation of that carbohydrate.

Table B-4
Comparison of Different Glycemic Loads

Source	Typical Volume	Glycemic Index	Glycemic Load
Pasta	1 cup	59	3,068
Apple	1	54	972
Broccoli	1 cup	50*	150

Estimated from the glycemic index of various boiled beans

Even though the glycemic index of each of these carbohydrates is about the same, 1 cup of pasta generates 20 times the insulin response of 1 cup of broccoli, and a single apple generates about 6 times the insulin response of 1 cup of broccoli. It is clear that the glycemic load based on the serving size of a carbohydrate is a much more valuable tool than the glycemic index. Table B-5, on pages 350–353, lists the glycemic loads of a wide variety of carbohydrates. For vegetables that have never been tested for their glycemic index, I have used an estimate of 50 (although it probably is considerably lower), as I did in Table B-4.

A good rule of thumb: Never consume a glycemic load of more than 3,000 in any one meal. As you can see from the data, if you are eating low-density carbohydrates, it is very difficult to have a meal with a high glycemic load. On the other hand, eating typical volumes of grain and other starch-based carbohydrates gives a meal a very high glycemic load and results in a far greater insulin response.

You can also understand why many of the carbohydrates found in traditional grain-based diets are likely to dramatically increase insulin levels. For example, white rice generates a tremendous amount of insulin response compared with the same volume of oatmeal or barley because rice has a greater glycemic load. Likewise, most breakfast cereals will have the same impact on insulin as a Snickers bar, since their glycemic loads are approximately the same. Meanwhile cooked vegetables represent a very low glycemic load, which is why they are a critical component of the Zone Diet.

Also remember that the more processed a food, the higher the glycemic load. This is why boiled beans have a much lower glycemic load than the same volume of canned beans. And when you make any bean (like black beans) into a soup, the glycemic load skyrockets because the prolonged cooking breaks down the cell walls of the bean, making it easier for the body to digest it into simple sugars for absorption.

Thus by using the concept of glycemic load it also becomes clear why consuming most of your carbohydrates from high-quality vegetables is the key to maintaining insulin levels within an appropriate zone.

Table B-5
Glycemic Loads of Various Tested Carbohydrates

Source	Typical Volume	Grams	Glycemic Index	Glycemic Load
Fruits				
Apple	1	18	54	972
Apple juice	8 oz	29	57	1,653
Apricot	1	4	81	324
Banana (medium)	1	32	79	2,528
Cantaloupe	1 cup	15	65	975
Cherries	10	10	31	310
Grapefruit	1	10	36	360
Grapefruit juice	8 oz	22	69	1,518
Grapes	1 cup	15	66	990
Kiwi	1	8	74	592
Mango (medium)	1	33	80	2,640
Orange (medium)	1	10	63	630
Orange juice	8 oz	26	66	1,716
Papaya (medium)	1	28	83	2,324
Peach	1	7	40	280
Pear	1	21	54	1,134
Plum	1	7	56	392
Raisins	1 cup	112	91	10,192
Watermelon	1 cup	11	103	1,133
Legumes				
Black beans (boiled)	1 cup	41	43	1,763
Black bean soup	1 cup	38	91	3,458
Chickpeas (boiled)	1 cup	46	47	2,162

Source	Typical Volume	Grams	Glycemic Index	Glycemic Load
Fava beans (boiled)	1 cup	34	113	3,978
Kidney beans (boiled)	1 cup	40	39	1,560
Kidney beans (canned)	1 cup	38	74	2,812
Lentils (boiled)	1 cup	32	43	1,376
Navy beans (boiled)	1 cup	38	54	2,052
Pinto beans (canned)	1 cup	36	64	2,304
Soy beans (boiled)	1 cup	20	26	520

Breads and Pasta

Source	Typical Volume	Grams	Glycemic Index	Glycemic Load
Bagel, small	1	38	103	3,914
Bread, dark rye	1 slice	18	109	1,962
Bread, sourdough	1 slice	20	74	1,480
Bread, white	1 slice	12	100	1,200
Bread, whole-wheat	1 slice	13	99	1,287
Croissant (medium)	1	27	96	2,592
Hamburger bun	1	22	86	1,892
Kaiser roll	1	34	104	3,536
Linguine	1 cup	56	79	4,424
Macaroni	1 cup	52	64	3,328
Pita bread	1	35	81	2,835
Pizza	1 slice	28	86	2,408
Spaghetti	1 cup	52	59	3,086

Source	Typical Volume	Grams	Glycemic Index	Glycemic Load
Starches, Grains, and Cereals				
Barley (boiled)	1 cup	44	36	1,584
Bulgur (cooked)	1 cup	31	69	2,139
Cheerios	1 cup	23	106	2,438
Corn, sweet (canned)	1 cup	30	79	2,370
Corn Chex	1 cup	26	119	3,094
Corn Flakes	1 cup	24	120	2,880
Couscous (cooked)	1 cup	42	93	3,906
Grape-Nuts	1 cup	108	96	10,368
Oatmeal (slow-cooking)	1 cup	24	70	1,680
Potato, white (baked)	1	24	121	2,904
Potato, white (boiled)	1	24	90	2,160
Potato, white (mashed)	1 cup	40	100	4,000
Rice, brown	1 cup	37	79	2,923
Rice, white	1 cup	42	103	4,326
Rice cakes	3	23	117	2,691
Rice Chex	1 cup	22	127	2,794
Rice Krispies	1 cup	21	117	2,457
Dairy Products				
Milk (low-fat)	1 cup	11	43	473
Soy milk	1 cup	14	44	616
Tofu, frozen	1 cup	42	164	6,888
Yogurt (plain)	1 cup	17	20	340

Source	Typical Volume	Grams	Glycemic Index	Glycemic Load

Vegetables (Cooked)

Source	Typical Volume	Grams	Glycemic Index	Glycemic Load
Artichoke hearts	1 cup	7	50*	350
Bok choy	1 cup	2	50*	100
Broccoli	1 cup	2	50*	100
Cabbage	1 cup	2	50*	100
Collard greens	1 cup	3	50*	150
Eggplant	1 cup	5	50*	250
Kale	1 cup	3	50*	150
Mushrooms	1 cup	3	50*	150
Onions	1 cup	14	50*	700
Spinach	1 cup	2	50*	150
String beans	1 cup	5	50*	250
Swiss chard	1 cup	4	50*	200
Zucchini	1 cup	4	50*	200

Others

Source	Typical Volume	Grams	Glycemic Index	Glycemic Load
Coca-Cola (regular)	1	39	90	3,510
Fructose	1 pck	3	33	100
Gatorade	8 oz	14	111	1,554
Granola bar	1	23	87	2,001
Honey	1 tbsp	16	83	1,328
Power Bar	1	45	83	3,735
Snickers bar	1	36	59	2,124
Table sugar	1 tsp	4	93	372

*Estimated glycemic index of 50

Appendix C

Using Zone Food Blocks for Making Zone Meals

Any long-term dietary program is simply an accounting system to keep track of your macronutrient balance. Some of these systems are based on counting calories during a given meal, or counting fat grams, or counting carbohydrates during the course of a day. Beyond a certain limit, you won't be successful in achieving your weight loss goal by using these techniques. The Zone Diet is based on a different concept—balance at every meal. You are trying to maintain a balance of protein to carbohydrate at each meal and snack to generate the appropriate hormonal response. If you get the right balance, you will lose excess body fat. In addition, you'll live longer and have a much lower risk of chronic disease.

The Zone Diet is like balancing your checkbook. You use your checkbook to track money coming in and money going out. You don't have to balance to the penny, but you do want to make sure you have enough money to write a check that won't bounce. Your diet is no different. You don't have to be obsessive, just have a general idea that you have a great enough hormonal balance so you don't bounce any hormonal checks in the next four to six hours. I believe the easiest way to balance your hormonal checkbook is by using the Zone Food Block method.

Remember that it is only the amount of insulin-stimulating carbohydrate in a meal that is important, which means that you have to subtract the fiber content of any carbohydrate. All of these calculations are done for you when you use Zone Food Blocks.

Similarly, only about 70 percent of the protein in vegetarian sources is absorbed because of the fiber content. The lower the fiber content, the higher the percentage of protein that is absorbed. Many of the soybean protein choices listed below are low in fiber, meaning that most of the protein will be absorbed.

Making Zone Meals simply requires balancing the number of protein, carbohydrate, and fat Zone Block servings in equal proportions. The typical female will need three Zone Blocks of *each* macronutrient at every meal, whereas the typical male will need four Zone Blocks of *each* macronutrient at every meal. Zone snacks consist of one Zone Block of *each* macronutrient. But again let me emphasize that you don't need to obsess over the exact amounts.

Thus for a typical female, each Zone meal would consist of three Zone Protein Blocks, three Zone Carbohydrate Blocks, and three Zone Fat Blocks. For the typical male, each meal would consist of four Zone Protein Blocks, four Zone Carbohydrate Blocks, and four Zone Fat Blocks. Feel free to mix and match the Zone Food Blocks within each macronutrient group as long as they add up pretty close to your required number of Zone Blocks at the end of the meal.

But be aware that many vegetarian protein sources tend to have associated carbohydrate blocks, so take this into account when constructing Zone meals.

ZONE PROTEIN BLOCKS

Each portion contains approximately 7 grams of absorbable protein per Zone Block.

Protein-Rich Sources	Per Zone Block	Zone Rating
Lobster	1½ oz	☺ ☺ ☺
Mackerel	1½ oz	☺ ☺ ☺
Salmon	1½ oz	☺ ☺ ☺
Scallops	1½ oz	☺ ☺ ☺
Trout	1½ oz	☺ ☺
Tuna	1½ oz	☺ ☺ ☺

Protein-Rich Sources	Per Zone Block	Zone Rating
Beef tenderloin	1 oz	☺
Chicken breast	1 oz	☺ ☺
Pork tenderloin	1 oz	☺
Protein powder	7 grams	☺ ☺ ☺
Sea bass	1½ oz	☺ ☺ ☺
Soybean Canadian bacon	3 slices	☺ ☺
Soybean frozen sausage	1 link	☺
Soybean hamburger crumbles	⅓ cup	☺ ☺ ☺
Soybean hot dog	1 link	☺
Tofu, extra-firm	2 oz	☺ ☺
Tofu, firm	3 oz	☺ ☺
Turkey breast	1 oz	☺ ☺ ☺

Mixed Protein Sources*	Per Zone Block	Associated Carb Blocks	Zone Rating
Milk, skim	6 oz	1	☺ ☺ ☺
Soy milk	8 oz	1	☺
Soybeans, boiled	⅓ cup	⅔	☺
Soybean hamburger	⅔ patty	⅓	☺ ☺
Tempeh	1½ oz	1	☺ ☺
Tofu, soft	4 oz	⅓	☺ ☺
Yogurt, skim	8 oz	1	☺ ☺

These contain more carbohydrates. Read the labels carefully.

ZONE CARBOHYDRATE BLOCKS

Each portion contains approximately 9 grams of insulin-stimulating carbohydrates per Zone Block.

Cooked Vegetables	Per Zone Block	Zone Rating
Artichoke	4 large	☺ ☺
Artichoke hearts	1 cup	☺ ☺
Asparagus	12 spears	☺ ☺
Beans, black	¼ cup	☺ ☺
Beans, green or wax	1½ cups	☺ ☺
Bok choy	3 cups	☺ ☺
Broccoli	3 cups	☺ ☺ ☺

Cooked Vegetables	Per Zone Block	Zone Rating
Brussels sprouts	1½ cups	😊 😊
Cabbage (red or green)	3 cups	😊 😊
Cauliflower	4 cups	😊 😊 😊
Chickpeas	¼ cup	😊
Collard greens, chopped	2 cups	😊 😊 😊
Eggplant	1½ cups	😊 😊
Kale	2 cups	😊 😊 😊
Kidney beans	¼ cup	😊
Leeks	1 cup	😊
Lentils	¼ cup	😊 😊
Mushrooms, whole, boiled	2 cups	😊
Okra, sliced	1 cup	😊 😊
Onions (all types), chopped, boiled	½ cup	😊
Spinach	3½ cups	😊 😊 😊
Squash, yellow, sliced, boiled	2 cups	😊
Swiss chard	2½ cups	😊 😊 😊
Tomato, canned, chopped	1 cup	😊 😊
Tomato puree	½ cup	😊 😊
Tomato sauce	½ cup	😊 😊
Turnip greens, chopped, boiled	4 cups	😊 😊 😊
Zucchini	2 cups	😊

Raw Vegetables	Per Zone Block	Zone Rating
Alfalfa sprouts	10 cups	☺☺☺
Bamboo shoots	4 cups	☺☺
Bean sprouts	3 cups	☺☺
Beans, green	2 cups	☺☺
Bell peppers (green or red)	2	☺☺
Broccoli	4 cups	☺☺☺
Brussels sprouts	1½ cups	☺☺
Cabbage, shredded	4 cups	☺☺
Cauliflower	4 cups	☺☺☺
Celery, sliced	2 cups	☺
Chickpeas	¼ cup	☺
Cucumber (medium)	1½	☺
Endive, chopped	10 cups	☺☺☺
Escarole, chopped	10 cups	☺☺☺
Jalapeño peppers	2 cups	☺
Lettuce, iceberg	2 heads	☺☺
Lettuce, romaine, shredded	10 cups	☺☺☺
Mushrooms, chopped	4 cups	☺
Onion, chopped	1 cup	☺☺
Radishes, sliced	4 cups	☺☺
Scallions	3 cups	☺
Shallots, diced	1½ cups	☺
Snow peas	1½ cups	☺☺

Raw Vegetables	Per Zone Block	Zone Rating
Spinach, chopped	20 cups	🙂 🙂 🙂
Tomato	2	🙂 🙂
Tomato, cherry	2 cups	🙂 🙂
Tomato, chopped	1½ cups	🙂 🙂

Fruits (Fresh, Frozen, or Canned Light)	Per Zone Block	Zone Rating
Apple	½	🙂
Applesauce (unsweetened)	⅓ cup	🙂
Apricots	3	🙂 🙂
Blackberries	¾ cup	🙂 🙂 🙂
Blueberries	½ cup	🙂 🙂 🙂
Boysenberries	½ cup	🙂 🙂 🙂
Cherries	8	🙂
Grapes	½ cup	🙂
Grapefruit	½	🙂 🙂
Kiwi	1	🙂 🙂
Nectarine	½	🙂 🙂
Orange	½	🙂
Orange, mandarin, canned in water	⅓ cup	🙂 🙂
Peach	1	🙂
Pear	½	🙂
Plum	1	🙂 🙂

Fruits (Fresh, Frozen, or Canned Light)	Per Zone Block	Zone Rating
Raspberries	1 cup	☺ ☺ ☺
Strawberries, diced fine	1 cup	☺ ☺ ☺

Grains	Per Zone Block	Zone Rating
Barley, dry	½ tablespoon	☺ ☺
Oatmeal, dry (slow cooking)	½ oz	☺ ☺
Oatmeal, cooked (slow cooking)	⅓ cup	☺ ☺

ZONE FAT BLOCKS

Each portion contains approximately 3 grams of fat per Zone Block.

Best (Rich in Monounsaturated Fats)	Per Zone Block	Zone Rating
Almond butter, natural	1 teaspoon	☺ ☺
Almond oil	⅔ teaspoon	☺ ☺
Almonds	6	☺ ☺
Avocado	2 tablespoons	☺ ☺
Canola oil	⅔ teaspoon	☺ ☺
Cashews	3	☺ ☺
Guacamole	2 tablespoons	☺ ☺
Macadamia nuts	2	☺ ☺ ☺

Best (Rich in Monounsaturated Fats)	Per Zone Block	Zone Rating
Olive oil	⅔ teaspoon	☺ ☺ ☺
Olives, black (medium)	5	☺ ☺ ☺
Peanuts	6	☺
Pistachios	3	☺ ☺

Zone Diet Validation Studies

The Zone Diet is perhaps the most misunderstood concept in nutritional research in the past five years. The Zone Diet is based upon controlling various hormones generated by the macronutrient (protein, carbohydrate, and fat) composition of each meal and keeping them within specified zones—not too high, not too low.

My first book, *The Zone*, outlined the biochemical rationale for the Zone Diet. However, since the publication of the revolutionary book, the Zone Diet has been incorrectly labeled as a high-protein diet. I'm always disappointed to hear it mentioned in the same breath as high-protein fad diets that bear no relationship to the Zone.

The Zone Diet is a protein-adequate, carbohydrate-moderate, low-fat diet. In fact, since the Zone Diet contains more carbohydrate than protein, it is hard to call it a high-protein diet. Furthermore, it is based on two principles: balance and moderation. You balance the protein, carbohydrate, and fat at each meal and consume only a moderate amount of calories at each meal.

The Zone Diet is neither a high-protein diet (too high in protein and too low in carbohydrate) nor a high-carbohydrate diet (too high in carbohydrate and too low in protein). In fact, the Zone Diet can be defined mathematically by the protein-to-carbohydrate ratio of a meal. That ratio is between 0.5 and 1.0. Below that ratio, you have a high-carbohydrate diet, and above that ratio you have a high-protein diet. Another way of describing the Zone Diet is that for every 1 gram of fat consumed at a meal, you should consume 2 grams of protein and 3 grams of carbohydrate. The fat component should be high quality—that is, rich in heart-healthy monounsaturated fat; the protein should be low-fat protein; and the carbohydrates should consist primarily of high-quality vegetables and fruits that are rich in anti-oxidants. What could be controversial about that?

I feel that the criticism surrounding the Zone Diet stems from the radical way it asks us to think about food. First, it asks us to consider the hormonal consequences of a meal and, in particular, to maintain the hormone insulin within a zone. This is a totally new concept to virtually everyone, including nutritionists and physicians. Second, the Zone Diet is based on the most recent advances in hormone research, of which many of its critics seem to be totally unaware.

Following, are some of the most recent independent studies that validate the Zone Diet. All of this research comes from reputable institutions, such as Harvard Medical School, and all the studies have been published in peer-reviewed research journals.

1. **The number-one risk factor that predicts heart disease is elevated insulin.** Prospective studies with individuals who show no sign of heart disease have

demonstrated that elevated insulin is a vastly more powerful predictor of future heart disease than cholesterol. In fact, elevated insulin increases the likelihood of having a heart attack by a factor of 5.5 compared with elevated "bad" (LDL) cholesterol, which only increased the likelihood by 2.4 times. Other prospective studies have indicated that the only blood factor associated with increased heart attacks is increased insulin. A case control study from Harvard Medical School has demonstrated that an elevated ratio of triglyceride-to-HDL cholesterol (an indirect marker of increased insulin levels) is 16 times more predictive of heart attacks than a low ratio. Other studies from Harvard Medical School also indicate that the higher the levels of insulin, the less likely the body is to dissolve clots that lead to heart attacks.

2. **The more protein you eat, the less likely you are to develop heart disease.** Recent long-term studies from Harvard Medical School indicate that there is a 26-percent decrease in heart disease when the ratio of protein to carbohydrate reaches the levels recommended by the Zone Diet. The group that had the lowest incidence of heart disease followed a diet that provided a protein-to-carbohydrate ratio of 0.7, squarely within the limits of the Zone Diet. A more recent analysis has indicated that if restriction of high-glycemic carbohydrates is factored in, the incidence of heart disease is reduced by nearly 50 percent.

3. **The more protein you eat, the fewer hip fractures you get.** In postmenopausal women, research has shown that increasing protein intake can reduce the number of hip fractures by 70 percent.

4. **The most powerful drug to prevent heart attacks is diet, as opposed to aspirin or any cholesterol-lowering drugs.** The Lyon Diet Heart Study indicated that a 65 percent reduction in both fatal and nonfatal heart attacks could be achieved simply by changing the balance of Omega-3 to Omega-6 polyunsaturated fats in the diet and by consuming more fruit. The decrease in both cardiovascular mortality and overall mortality following this diet was far greater than with aspirin or any other cholesterol-lowering drug. The Zone Diet is similar to the diet used in the Lyon Diet Heart Study except that the Zone Diet emphasizes an even greater intake of fruits and vegetables and puts an even greater emphasis on switching from Omega-6 to Omega-3 fatty acids.

5. **Increased dietary protein is associated with increased breast cancer survival.** As long as you decrease your consumption of red meat, you will be more likely to survive breast cancer if you increase your consumption of protein. The protein recommendation of the Zone Diet is consistent with this study.

6. **Increasing monounsaturated fat and decreasing carbohydrate is healthier than the diet recommended by the American Heart Association.** That was the conclusion of a recent study directly comparing a diet rich in monounsaturated fat with that proposed by the American Heart Association. The authors state that "it is now timely to reevaluate what the optimal diet is for lowering risk of cardiovascular disease." The Zone Diet is rich in monounsaturated fat with a decreased carbohydrate content and thus should be considered the future standard for treatment and prevention of cardiovascular disease.

7. **You lose body fat faster on the Zone Diet.** In fact, fat loss is nearly twice as great on the Zone Diet than on a higher-carbohydrate diet, even though both diets contain the same number of calories and the same amount of fat. In addition, it has been shown that the Zone Diet reduces both cholesterol and triglyceride levels in normal individuals to a greater extent than other low-calorie diets with the same amount of fat but greater levels of carbohydrate.

8. **The Zone Diet can improve your hormone levels in only one meal.** This was confirmed by research conducted at Harvard Medical School with overweight adolescents. The Zone meal generated a completely different hormonal profile than a standard meal, even though both contained the same number of calories. Furthermore, after a Zone meal the number of calories consumed at the next meal was significantly less, indicating that the Zone Diet provides better hunger control. The same researchers at Harvard Medical School have recently demonstrated that within six days on the Zone Diet, you get a significant metabolism boost.

9. **The Zone Diet can reduce excess insulin levels before any fat loss is achieved.** This study helps answer the chicken and egg question: which comes first, elevated insulin or increased body fat? Elevated insulin levels were lowered far before any fat loss was achieved, thus confirming earlier research demonstrating that elevated insulin levels occur before the accumulation of body fat. More important, the underlying cause of Type 2 diabetes and obesity (insulin resistance) was reversed within four days on the Zone Diet. No drug can work that quickly (and, of course, the Zone Diet has no side effects).

10. **The Zone Diet can alter your genetic code.** It has been known for more than 60 years that calorie-restricted diets extend longevity. Recently it has been shown that calorie-restricted programs can also alter the expression of the genetic code. The Zone Diet is a calorie-restricted diet that supplies adequate protein, adequate essential fat, a moderate amount of carbohydrate, adequate levels of vitamins and minerals, and is guaranteed to reverse aging but without hunger or deprivation since blood sugar levels are maintained.

References

INTRODUCTION

Sears, Barry. *The Zone*. New York: Regan Books, 1995.

CHAPTER 1 MAKING THE TOP 100

Holmes, M. D., M. J. Stampfer, Rosner B. Colditz, D. J. Hunter, and W. C. Willett. "Dietary factors and the survival of women with breast cancer." *Cancer* 86:751–753 (1999).

Lamarche, B., A. Tchernot, P. Mauriege, B. Cantin, P.-J. Lupien, and J.-P. Depres. "Fasting insulin and apolipoprotein B levels and low density particle size as risk factors for ischemic heart disease." *Journal of the American Medical Association* 279:1955–1961 (1998).

Markovic, T. P., A. B. Jenkins, L. V. Campbell, S. M. Furler, E. W. Kraegen, and D. J. Chisholm. "The determinants of glycemic responses to diet restriction and weight loss in obesity and NIDDM." *Diabetes Care* 21:687–694 (1998).

Munger, R. G., J. R. Cerhan, and B. C.-H. Chiu. "Prospective study of dietary protein intake and risk of hip fracture in postmenopausal women." *American Journal of Clinical Nutrition* 69:147–152 (1999).

CHAPTER 2 YOUR ZONE PRIMER

Ascherio, A., M. B. Katan, P. L. Zock, M. J. Stampfer, and W. C. Willett. "Trans fatty acids and coronary heart disease." *New England Journal of Medicine* 340:1994–1998 (1999).

Sears, Barry. *The Anti-Aging Zone*. New York: Regan Books, 1999.

———. *The Soy Zone*. New York: Regan Books, 2000.

CHAPTER 3 THE HEALTHIEST FOODS IN THE WORLD

Cao, G., E. Sofic, and R. L. Prior. "Antioxidant capacity of tea and common vegetables." *Journal of Agricultural and Food Chemistry* 44:3426–3431 (1996).

Prior, R.L., and G. Cao. "Antioxidant capacity as influenced by total phenolic and anthocyanin content, maturity, and variety of vaccinium species." *Journal of Agricultural and Food Chemistry* 46:2686–2693 (1998).

Sears, Barry. *The Zone*. New York: Regan Books, 1995.

Steinmetz, K. A., and J. D. Potter. "Vegetables, fruit, and cancer prevention: a review." *Journal of the American Dietetic Association* 96:1027–1039 (1996).

Wang, H., G. Cao, and R.L. Prior. "Total antioxidant capacity of fruits." *Journal of Agricultural and Food Chemistry* 44:701–705 (1996).

Willett, W. C. "Diet and health: what should we eat?" *Science* 264:532–537 (1994).

Verlangieri, A. J., J. C. Kapeghian, S. el-Dean, and M. Bush. "Fruit and vegetable consumption and cardiovascular mortality." *Medical Hypotheses* 16:7–15 (1985).

CHAPTER 4 THE TOP 100 ZONE FOODS

Applegate, L. *How to Eat Away Heart Disease and High Blood Pressure*. Paramus, N.J.: Prentice Hall, 1999.

Carper, J. *The Food Pharmacy*. New York: Bantam Books, 1988.

Jensen, B. *Foods That Heal*. Garden City Park, N.Y.: Avery, 1993.

Mindell, E. *Earl Mindell's Food as Medicine*. New York: Fireside, 1994.

Reader's Digest. *Foods That Harm, Foods That Heal*. Pleasantville, N.Y.: Reader's Digest Association, 1997.

CHAPTER 6 ZONE SUPPLEMENTS

Adams, P. B., S. Lawson, A. Sanigorski, and A. J. Sinclair. "Arachidonic acid to eicosapentaenoic acid ratio in blood correlates positively with clinical symptoms of depression." *Lipids* 31:S157–161 (1996).

Eades, M. D. *The Doctor's Complete Guide to Vitamins and Minerals*. New York: Dell Publishing, 1994.

Lanting, C. I., V. Fidler, M. Huisman, B. C. L. Touwen, and E. R. Boersma. "Neurological differences between 9-year-old children fed breast-milk or formula-milk as babies." *Lancet* 344:1319–1322 (1994).

Rimm, E. B., M. J. Stampfer, A. Ascheriom, E. Giovannucci, G. A. Golditz, and W. C. Willett. "Vitamin E consumption and risk of coronary heart disease in

men." *New England Journal of Medicine*
328:1450–1456 (1993).

Stampfer, M. J., C. H. Hennekens, J. E. Manson,
G. A. Coditz, B. Rosner, and W. C. Willett. "Vitamin E consumption and risk of coronary heart disease in women." *New England Journal of Medicine*
328:1444–1449 (1993).

Stevens, L. J., S. Zentall, and J. R. Burgress. "Omega-3
fatty acids in boys with behavior, learning, and
health problems." *Physiology and Behavior*
59:915–920 (1996).

Stevens, L. J., S. Zentall, J. L. Deck, M. L. Abate, B. A.
Watkins, S. R. Lipp, and J. R. Burgress. "Essential
fatty acid metabolism in boys with attention-deficit
hyperactivity disorder." *American Journal of Clinical Nutrition* 62:761–768 (1995).

Stoll, A. L., E. Severus, M. P. Freeman, S. Rueter, H. A.
Zhoyan, E. Diamond, K. K. Cress, and L. B.
Marangell. "Omega-3 fatty acids in bipolar disorder."
Archives of General Psychiatry 56:407–412 (1999).

CHAPTER 7 FOOD AND HORMONES

Markovic, T. P., A. B. Jenkins, L. V. Campbell, S. M.
Furler, E. W. Kraegen, and D. J. Chisholm. "The
determinants of glycemic responses to diet restriction and weight loss in obesity and NIDDM." *Diabetes Care* 21:687–694 (1998).

Sears, Barry. *The Anti-Aging Zone*. New York: Regan
Books, 1999.

———. *The Soy Zone*. New York: Regan Books, 2000.

———. *The Zone*. New York: Regan Books, 1995.

Unger, R. H. "Glucagon and the insulin: glucagon ratio
in diabetes and other catabolic illnesses." *Diabetes*
20:834–838 (1971).

Unger, R. H., and P. J. Lefebvre. *Glucagon: Molecular Physiology, Clinical and Therapeutic Implications.* Oxford: Pergamon Press, 1972.

CHAPTER 8 THE ZONE VS. OTHER DIETS

Depres, J.-P., B. Lamarche, P. Mauriege, B. Cantin, G. R. Dagenais, S. Moorjani, and P.-J. Lupien. "Hyperinsulinemia as an independent risk factor for ischemic heart disease." *New England Journal of Medicine* 334:952–957 (1996).

De Lorgeril, M., P. Salen, J.-L. Martin, I. Monjaud, J. Delaye, and N. Mamelle. "Mediterranean diet, traditional risk factors, and rate of cardiovascular complications after myocardial infarction. Final report of the Lyon Diet Heart Study." *Circulation* 99:779–785 (1999).

Jain, S. K., K. Kannan, and G. Lim. "Ketosis (acetoacetate) can generate oxygen radicals and cause increased lipid peroxidation and growth inhibition in human endothelial cells." *Free Radical Biology and Medicine* 25:1083–1088 (1998).

Jain, S. K., and R. McVie. "Hyperketonemia can increase lipid peroxidation and lower glutathione levels in human erthrocytes in vitro and in Type 1 diabetic patients." *Diabetes* 48:1850–1855 (1999).

Jain, S. K., R. McVie, R. Jackson, S. N. Levine, and G. Lim. "Effect of hyperketonemia on plasma lipid peroxidation levels in diabetic patients." *Diabetes Care* 22:1171–1175 (1999).

Lichenstein, A. H., and L. VanHorn, "Very Low Fat Diets." *Circulation* 98:935-939 (1998).

Ornish, D., L. W. Scherwitz, J. H. Billings, K. L. Gould, T. A. Merritt, S. Sparler, W. T. Armstrong, T. A. Ports, R. L. Kirkeeide, C. Hogeboom, and R. J.

Brand. "Intensive lifestyle changes for reversal of coronary heart disease." *Journal of the American Medical Association* 280:2001–2007 (1998).

APPENDIX D ZONE DIET VALIDATION STUDIES

Agus, M. S. D., J. F. Swain, C. L. Larson, E. A. Eckert, and D. S. Ludwig. "Dietary composition and physiologic adaptations to energy restriction." *American Journal of Clinical Nutrition* 71:901–907 (2000).

Boyko, E. J., D. L. Leonetti, R. W. Bergestrom, L. Newell-Morris, and W. Y. Fujimoto. "Low insulin secretion and high fasting insulin and C-peptide predict increased visceral adiposity." *Diabetes* 45:1010–1015 (1996).

De Lorgeril, M., P. Salen, J.-L. Martin, I. Monjaud, J. Delaye, and N. Mamelle. "Mediterranean diet, traditional risk factors, and rate of cardiovascular complications after myocardial infarction. Final report of the Lyon Diet Heart Study." *Circulation* 99:779–785 (1999).

Depres, J.-P., B. Lamarche, P. Mauriege, B. Cantin, G. R. Dagenais, S. Moorjani, and P.-J. Lupien. "Hyperinsulinemia as an independent risk factor for ischemic heart disease." *New England Journal of Medicine* 334:952–957 (1996).

Gaziano, J. M., C. H. Hennekens, C. H. O'Donnell, J. L. Breslow, and J. E. Buring. "Fasting triglycerides, high-density lipoproteins, and risk of myocardial infarction." *Circulation* 96:2520–2525 (1997).

Holmes, M. D., M. J. Stampfer, Rosner B. Colditz, D. J. Hunter, and W. C. Willett. "Dietary factors and the survival of women with breast cancer." *Cancer* 86:751–753 (1999).

Hu, F. B., M. J. Stampfer, J. E. Manson, E. Rimm, G. A. Colditz, F. E. Speizer, C. H. Hennekens, and W. C. Willett. "Dietary protein and the risk of ischemic heart disease in women." *American Journal of Clinical Nutrition* 70:221–227 (1999).

Kris-Etherton, P. M., T. A. Pearson, Y. Wan, R. L. Hargrove, K. Moriaty, V. Fishell, and T. D. Etherton. "High-monounsaturated fatty acid diets lower both plasma cholesterol and triacylglycerol concentrations." *American Journal of Clinical Nutrition* 70:1009–1015 (1999).

Lamarche, B., A. Tchernot, P. Mauriege, B. Cantin, P.-J. Lupien, and J.-P. Depres. "Fasting insulin and apolipoprotein B levels and low density particle size as risk factors for ischemic heart disease." *Journal of the American Medical Association* 279:1955–1961 (1998).

Lee, C.-K., R. G. Klopp, R. Weindruch, and T. A. Prolla. "Gene expression profile of aging and its retardation by caloric restriction." *Science* 285:1390–1393 (1999).

Liu, S., W. C. Willett, M. J. Stampfer, F. B. Hu, M. Franz, L. Sampson, C. H. Hennekens, and J. E. Manson. "A prospective study of dietary glycemic load, carbohydrate intake, and risk of coronary heart disease in U.S. women." *American Journal of Clinical Nutrition* 71:1455–1461 (2000).

Ludwig, D. S., J. A. Majzoub, A. Al-Zahrani, G. E. Dallal, I. Blanco, and S. B. Roberts. "High glycemic index foods, overeating, and obesity." *Pediatrics* 103:E26 (1999).

Markovic, T. P., A. B. Jenkins, L. V. Campbell, S. M. Furler, E. W. Kraegen, and D. J. Chisholm. "The determinants of glycemic responses to diet restriction and weight loss in obesity and NIDDM." *Diabetes Care* 21:687–694 (1998).

Meigs, J. B., M. A. Mittleman, D. M. Nathan, G. H. Tofler, D. E. Singer, P. M. Murphy-Sheehy, I. Lipinska, R. B. D'Agostino, and P. W. F. Wilson. "Hyperinsulinemia, hyperglycemia, and impaired hemostasis." *Journal of the American Medical Association* 283:221–228 (2000).

Munger, R. G., J. R. Cerhan, and B. C.-H. Chiu. "Prospective study of dietary protein intake and risk of hip fracture in postmenopausal women." *American Journal of Clinical Nutrition* 69:147–152 (1999).

Odeleye, O. D., M. de Courten, D. J. Pettit, and E. Ravassin. "Fasting hyperinsulinemia is a predictor of increased body weight gain and obesity in Pima Indian children." *Diabetes* 46:1341–1345 (1997).

Scandinavian Simvastatin Survival Study Group. "Randomized trial of cholesterol lowering in 4444 patients with coronary heart disease: the Scandinavian Simvastatin Survival Study (4S)." *Lancet* 344:1383–1389 (1994).

Skov, A. R., S. Toubro, B. Ronn, L. Holm, and A. Astrup. "Randomized trial on protein vs carbohydrate in ad libitum fat reduced diet for the treatment of obesity." *International Journal of Obesity* 23:528–536 (1999).

Steering Committee of the Physician Health Study Research Group. "Preliminary report findings from the aspirin component of the ongoing Physician Health Study." *New England Journal of Medicine* 320:262–264 (1988).

Wolfe, B. M. J., and L. A. Piche. "Replacement of carbohydrate by protein in a conventional-fat diet reduces cholesterol and triglyceride concentrations in healthy normolipidemic subjects." *Clinical and Investigative Medicine* 22:140–148 (1999).

Index